Unhealthy Alcohol Use in Older Adults

About the Author

Erin L. Woodhead, PhD, is associate professor of psychology at San José State University, California. She is a licensed psychologist who has published over 30 journal articles in the areas of substance use, mental health, and aging, as well as an edited textbook entitled *Psychology of Aging*. She teaches courses in clinical psychology, adult psychopathology, psychology of aging, addictions, and lifespan development.

Erin L. Woodhead

Unhealthy Alcohol Use in Older Adults

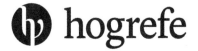

Library of Congress Cataloging in Publication information for the print version of this book is available via the Library of Congress Marc Database under the LC Control Number 2023939163

Library and Archives Canada Cataloguing in Publication
Title: Unhealthy alcohol use in older adults / Erin L. Woodhead.
Names: Woodhead, Erin L., author.
Description: Includes bibliographical references.
Identifiers: Canadiana (print) 20230467679 | Canadiana (ebook) 20230467741 | ISBN 9780889375109 (softcover) | ISBN 9781616765101 (PDF) | ISBN 9781613345108 (EPUB)
Subjects: LCSH: Older people—Alcohol use. | LCSH: Alcoholism—Treatment.
Classification: LCC HV5138 .W66 2023 | DDC 362.292/80846—dc23

© 2024 by Hogrefe Publishing
http://www.hogrefe.com

Cover image: © miodrag ignjatovic – iStock.com

The authors and publisher have made every effort to ensure that the information contained in this text is in accord with the current state of scientific knowledge, recommendations, and practice at the time of publication. In spite of this diligence, errors cannot be completely excluded. Also, due to changing regulations and continuing research, information may become outdated at any point. The authors and publisher disclaim any responsibility for any consequences which may follow from the use of information presented in this book.

Registered trademarks are not noted specifically as such in this publication. The use of descriptive names, registered names, and trademarks does not imply, even in the absence of a specific statement, that such names are exempt from the relevant protective laws and regulations and therefore free for general use.

PUBLISHING OFFICES
USA: Hogrefe Publishing Corporation, 44 Merrimac St., Suite 207, Newburyport, MA 01950
Phone (978) 255 3700; E-mail customersupport@hogrefe.com
EUROPE: Hogrefe Publishing GmbH, Merkelstr. 3, 37085 Göttingen, Germany
Phone +49 551 99950-0, Fax +49 551 99950-111; E-mail publishing@hogrefe.com
SALES & DISTRIBUTION
USA: Hogrefe Publishing, Customer Services Department,
30 Amberwood Parkway, Ashland, OH 44805
Phone (800) 228-3749, Fax (419) 281-6883; E-mail customersupport@hogrefe.com
UK: Hogrefe Publishing, c/o Marston Book Services Ltd., 160 Eastern Ave., Milton Park, Abingdon, OX14 4SB
Phone +44 1235 465577, Fax +44 1235 465556; E-mail direct.orders@marston.co.uk
EUROPE: Hogrefe Publishing, Merkelstr. 3, 37085 Göttingen, Germany
Phone +49 551 99950-0, Fax +49 551 99950-111; E-mail publishing@hogrefe.com
OTHER OFFICES
CANADA: Hogrefe Publishing, 82 Laird Drive, East York, Ontario, M4G 3V1
SWITZERLAND: Hogrefe Publishing, Länggass-Strasse 76, 3012 Bern

No part of this book may be reproduced, stored in a retrieval system or transmitted, in any form or by any means, electronic, mechanical, photocopying, microfilming, recording or otherwise, without written permission from the publisher.

Printed and bound in the USA

ISBN 978-0-88937-510-9 (print) · ISBN 978-1-61676-510-1 (PDF) · ISBN 978-1-61334-510-8 (EPUB)
https://doi.org/10.1027/00510-000

Acknowledgments

I would like to thank Jennifer K. Manuel, PhD, and Derek D. Satre, PhD, who spent a significant amount of time on earlier versions of this book, providing edits and content for the clinical cases and clinical pearls throughout the book. I would also like to thank my mentors throughout my career, including Steven Zarit, PhD, Barry Edelstein, PhD, and Christine Timko, PhD. Dr. Timko encouraged my interest in substance use research and continues to be an invaluable mentor. I am also appreciative of my colleagues at San José State University and the students who were part of my research lab while I was working on this book.

Erin L. Woodhead, PhD

Table of Contents

Acknowledgments		V
1	**Introduction**	1
1.1	Defining Older Adulthood	2
2	**Prevalence and Risk Factors**	3
2.1	Common Terms to Describe Alcohol Use	3
2.2	Prevalence of Unhealthy Alcohol Use Among Older Adults	6
2.2.1	Prevalence of Unhealthy Alcohol Use Among Racial and Ethnic Minority Older Adults	7
2.2.2	International Studies on Prevalence of Unhealthy Alcohol Use Among Older Adults	8
2.2.3	Prevalence of Unhealthy Alcohol Use Among Sexual and Gender Minority Older Adults	9
2.2.4	Prevalence Conclusions	9
2.3	Comorbid Nicotine and Other Drug Use	10
2.4	Conclusions: Prevalence and Risk Factors	11
3	**Conceptualizing Unhealthy Alcohol Use Among Older Adults**	12
3.1	Age-Related Changes in Alcohol Processing	12
3.2	Early Versus Late Onset	13
3.3	Life Transitions and Unhealthy Alcohol Use	15
3.4	Biopsychosocial Model	16
3.5	Stress and Coping Framework	18
3.6	Cognitive Behavioral Model	20
3.7	Conclusions: Conceptualizing Unhealthy Alcohol Use	22
4	**Diagnosing Unhealthy Alcohol Use Among Older Adults**	23
4.1	DSM-5 Criteria for Alcohol Use Disorder	23
4.2	Identification of Unhealthy Alcohol Use and Diagnosis	25
4.2.1	Common Signs of Unhealthy Alcohol Use	26
4.3	Differential Diagnoses to Consider	26
4.3.1	Cognitive Changes With Age	29
4.3.2	Long-Term Alcohol Use and Cognitive Impairment	30
4.4	Comorbid Medical and Mental Health Conditions	31
4.4.1	Comorbid Mental Health Conditions	31
4.5	Conclusions: Diagnosing Unhealthy Alcohol Use	33

VIII   Table of Contents

5	**Screening and Assessment**	34
5.1	Screening Recommendations	35
5.2	Assessment of Unhealthy Alcohol Use	38
5.2.1	Assessing Medically Complex Older Adults	39
5.3	Choosing Appropriate Assessment Tools	40
5.3.1	Alcohol Use Disorders Identification Test	41
5.3.2	Michigan Alcoholism Screening Test – Geriatric Version – and Short MAST-G	42
5.4	Conclusions: Screening and Assessment of Unhealthy Alcohol Use	42
6	**Psychological Interventions**	44
6.1	Care Coordination	45
6.2	Treatment Modifications for Older Adults	46
6.3	Harm Reduction Versus Abstinence-Based Treatments	48
6.4	Brief Interventions	49
6.5	Motivational Interviewing	51
6.6	Cognitive Behavioral Therapy	58
6.7	Mutual Help Groups	69
6.8	Family-Involved Treatments	72
6.9	Effectiveness of Treatments for Unhealthy Alcohol Use Among Older Adults	73
6.10	Conclusions: Psychological Interventions for Unhealthy Alcohol Use	78
7	**Pharmacological Interventions**	79
7.1	Disulfiram	79
7.2	Naltrexone	80
7.3	Acamprosate	80
7.4	Integrating Pharmacotherapy With Psychotherapy	81
7.5	Conclusions: Pharmacological Interventions	81
8	**Cultural Adaptations**	82
8.1	Cultural Adaptations to Treatment	82
8.2	Treatment Considerations for Sexual and Gender Minority Older Adults	84
8.3	Treatment Considerations for Older Women	86
8.4	Conclusions: Cultural Adaptations	87
9	**General Conclusions**	89
10	**Further Reading**	90
References		91

Notes on Supplementary Materials 103
Patient Health Questionnaire-9 (PHQ-9)............................. 104
Generalized Anxiety Disorder Screener (GAD-7) 106
Alcohol Use Disorders Identification Test – Consumption (AUDIT-C)...... 107
Short Michigan Alcoholism Screening Test – Geriatric Version
(SMAST-G) 108

1

Introduction

The proportion of older adults in the US population is increasing. Demographic trends indicate that by 2030, about 21% of the US population will be 65 or older, compared with 16% in 2019 (Administration of Community Living, 2021). This trend is also reflected internationally. In 2030, one in six individuals globally will be 60 years or older. Between 2020 and 2050, the world's population of older adults is expected to double from 1 billion to 2.1 billion (World Health Organization, 2022). As the population of older adults grows, so does concern about the impact of unhealthy alcohol use in this population.

This book highlights the unique concerns related to unhealthy alcohol use among older adults, and the clinical implications of the presented research. This book is intended for practitioners who are looking to expand their practice in this area, either toward expanding their work with older adults to include unhealthy alcohol use, or expanding work in the area of substance use to include older adults. Recommendations are offered throughout the book for ways to adapt diagnosis, assessment, and treatment to older adults; however, all of the recommendations need to be considered in the context of the individual client. Although older adults tend to be considered as one homogenous group, there are many differences between older adults, particularly those born in different generations. Some older clients may need treatment modifications to account for age-related cognitive changes, though caution is needed in assuming that all older adults need similar modifications.

This book offers a lifespan approach to understanding unhealthy alcohol use among older adults – that is, there are predictable shifts in alcohol use across the lifespan (Lee & Sher, 2018), particularly around common transitions points such as parenting and employment. Younger adults (ages 18–29) have the highest prevalence of drinking and alcohol-related problems (Barry & Blow, 2016). As individuals get older and gain more career and family-related responsibilities, they often reduce their alcohol consumption. Others, however, continue to drink at levels that put them at risk for health and psychosocial problems. For some groups, particularly women, new patterns of unhealthy alcohol use may emerge in middle age or later in life. These trends contribute to the increasing importance of better understanding unhealthy alcohol use among older adults, as well as appropriate psychological interventions.

This book reviews the prevalence of alcohol use among older adults, ways to conceptualize alcohol use among older adults, diagnostic considerations for alcohol use disorder among older adults, screening and assessment options, and treatment considerations relevant to health care and social service providers. Chapter 2 starts by summarizing the continuum of alcohol use, as well as epidemiological data on alcohol use among older adults. Chapter 3 presents common ways to conceptualize unhealthy alcohol use among older adults. Chapter 4 focuses on the diagnosis of alcohol use disorder among older adults, what to consider in the differential diagnosis of unhealthy alcohol use among older adults, and common comorbid conditions among older adults. Following this, recommendations for screening and assessing alcohol use among older adults are presented in Chapter 5. Chapter 6 describes psychological interventions, with a specific focus on how to consider lifespan development when providing care, as well as the relevance of common life transitions and generational differences. Case examples are used to demonstrate intervention approaches across a range of problem severity, highlighting treatment considerations relevant to health care professionals working with older adults. Chapter 7 provides a brief overview of pharmacological interventions. Finally, the role of culture in treatment, including race/ethnicity, gender, and sexual orientation are reviewed.

This book addresses problems with alcohol use specifically. Although use of other drugs, particularly cannabis, appears to be increasing among older adults (Han & Palamar, 2020), alcohol remains by far the most commonly used and most problematic substance in this age group. When relevant, however, treatment considerations applicable to managing other comorbid substance use problems are noted.

1.1 Defining Older Adulthood

For the purposes of this book, the general assumption is that "older adult" is defined as a person aged 65 and older. It is worth noting, however, that the literature on alcohol use among older adults varies with regard to what age is used as a cutoff for older adulthood. Some studies of alcohol use among older adults use a cutoff of age 55 or older (French et al., 2014; Gell et al., 2015). The rationale for using a younger cutoff is related to the mortality hypothesis, which is that individuals with more severe alcohol use may die younger and therefore may not live to age 65 years or older. Additionally, there is the belief that chronic alcohol use ages individuals prematurely, therefore contributing to a need to expand the definition of older adulthood to a include a slightly younger age range. Throughout the book, studies that defined older adults to include ages younger than 65 are noted.

2

Prevalence and Risk Factors

This chapter reviews the prevalence of *alcohol use disorder* (AUD) and unhealthy alcohol use, as well as differences by generation or birth cohort, gender, race/ethnicity, and sexual and gender minority status. Before reviewing data on prevalence rates, it is important to define what is meant by *unhealthy alcohol use* and briefly review what is meant by a standard drink.

2.1   Common Terms to Describe Alcohol Use

Alcohol use occurs on a continuum ranging from low-risk or nonproblematic use, to substantial consequences that warrant an AUD diagnosis (Saitz, 2005). Many terms are used in the literature to describe the continuum of alcohol use, including:

- *Low-risk drinking:* Patterns of use that fall below the recommended guidelines (for women, no more than three drinks on any 1 day and no more than seven drinks per week; for men, no more than four drinks per day and 14 drinks per week). This level of drinking typically does not meet criteria for an AUD diagnosis.
- *Risky drinking:* Patterns of use that increase the chances of having adverse consequences. This level of drinking may meet criteria for an AUD diagnosis.
- *Problem drinking* or *hazardous drinking:* A pattern of drinking that results in problems such as financial, health, or social consequences. This level of drinking typically does meet criteria for an AUD diagnosis.
- *Binge drinking:* Alcohol use within a short amount of time, which results in elevated blood alcohol content (BAC) of 0.08 g/dl or above (National Institute on Alcohol Abuse and Alcoholism [NIAAA], 2021). This level of drinking typically does meet criteria for an AUD diagnosis.

The National Institute on Drug Abuse (NIDA) recommends that practitioners avoid the use of stigmatizing terms when talking about substance use (see Kelly et al., 2016). As an example, "hazardous alcohol use" is preferred over "alcohol abuse," which may be an adjustment for practitioners trained under the *Diagnostic and Statistical Manual of Mental Disorders*, 4th edition (DSM-IV), when the terms "abuse" and "dependence" were more commonly used in clinical settings. In addition, terms such as "addict," "alcoholic," and "substance abuser," have negative connotations. A descriptor such as "older adult with hazardous alcohol use" is preferable. This book uses the term "unhealthy alcohol use" as defined by Saitz (2005), including risky drinking and extending to severe AUDs.

Table 1 demonstrates the continuum of alcohol use ranging from abstinence to severe AUD. Defining different levels of alcohol use informs studies on the prevalence of alcohol use among older adults, and can inform the selection of an appropriate level of intervention. For example, the intensity of an intervention may vary depending on the individual's drinking severity. Thus, defining alcohol use on a continuum can facilitate the selection of an appropriate level of intervention.

Table 1.   Alcohol use occurs on a continuum. Adapted from Saitz (2005).

	Abstinence	Low-risk drinking	Risky use	Problem drinking	Severe AUD
Common definition	No current alcohol use	For women, no more than three drinks in a day and no more than seven drinks per week. For men, no more than four drinks in a day and no more than 14 drinks per week.	Drinking above the low-risk guidelines, with no consequences currently occurring. This level of drinking puts individuals at risk for adverse consequences in the future.	Drinking above the guidelines with consequences in one or more areas. May meet criteria for a mild or moderate AUD.	Six or more DSM-5 criteria met for AUD

Note. AUD = alcohol use disorder.

Unhealthy alcohol use can range from risky drinking to diagnosable conditions including AUDs (Saitz, 2005). NIAAA recommends that men limit their alcohol consumption to no more than four drinks on any 1 day and to no more than 14 drinks per week, whereas the recommendation for women is no more than three drinks per day and no more than seven drinks per week (NIAAA, 2018). Any amount less than this is considered low-risk drinking. Drinking greater amounts of alcohol increases the risk for significant health, social, and legal consequences. The 2020–2025 Dietary Guidelines for Americans differ from the low-risk drinking guidelines offered by the NIAAA, suggesting that adults limit their daily alcohol intake to two drinks or fewer for men and one drink or fewer for women (US Department of Agriculture and US Department of Health and Human Services, 2020).

Internationally, countries differ on cutoffs for recommended drinking limits (Kerr & Stockwell, 2012). The UK guidelines recommend that adults limit their drinking to no more than 14 standard drinks in a week. Australia's recommendation is to limit drinking to no more than two standard drinks per day. Unlike the US, these countries do not differentiate between drinking limits for men and women, though other countries do. For example, Ireland's guidelines suggest no more than 17 standard drinks per week for men and 11 for women. This information is included here to note the variability both within the US and internationally, about recommended alcohol limits.

In the US, a standard drink is one that contains about 14 g of pure alcohol. This corresponds roughly to a 12-oz can of beer, a 5-oz glass of wine, or a 1.5-oz shot of liquor. The concept of a standard drink is meant to help estimate the alcohol content of different drink concentrations and serving sizes. It is important to note that the definition of a standard drink varies by country. For example, a standard drink in the UK is one that contains about 8 g of pure alcohol, whereas the definition in Ireland is 10 g of pure alcohol. It can thus be challenging to estimate the number of drinks accurately, since serving sizes and alcohol concentrations vary substantially (e.g., alcohol content in beer has increased in recent years). Many practitioners find it useful to use a visual aid such as a laminated card that illustrates what a standard drink is for different types of alcoholic beverages (see example in Table 2).

Table 2. Standard drink equivalents. Adapted from the National Institute on Alcohol Abuse and Alcoholism (2018).

Drink type and standard size	Typical alcohol content	Approximate number of standard drinks
Beer or cooler (12 oz)	~5%	12 oz = 1 16 oz = 1.3 22 oz = 2 40 oz = 3.3
Malt liquor (8–9 oz)	~7%	12 oz = 1.5 16 oz = 2 22 oz = 2.5 40 oz = 4.5
Table wine (5 oz)	~12%	25-oz bottle = 5
80-proof distilled spirits (1.5 oz)	~40%	A mixed drink = 1 or more A pint (16 oz) = 11 A fifth (25 oz) = 17 1.75 L (59 oz) = 39

Note. Standard drink amounts may not reflect customary serving sizes. Alcohol concentrations also vary significantly by brand.

2.2 Prevalence of Unhealthy Alcohol Use Among Older Adults

This section presents the prevalence of AUDs and unhealthy alcohol use among older adults, as well as differences by generation or birth cohort, gender, race/ethnicity, and sexual and gender minority status. Also presented are the prevalence rates for nicotine and other drugs among older adults, since use of multiple substances is common (Crummy et al., 2020). Each generation, or birth cohort, has its own set of values and characteristics depending on larger societal conditions at the time of their childhood and entrance into adulthood. Although these generational characteristics are certainly not consistent across all individuals, the classification of specific birth cohorts and their traits has been used to understand broad differences in alcohol use norms, preferences, and attitudes (Slade et al., 2016). As each generation gets older, they bring with them a certain set of values and experiences typical of their generation, which may continue to influence their behavior during older adulthood. These values and experiences impact a range of health behaviors including diet, exercise, alcohol, smoking, and use of other substances.

Understanding the substance use patterns of each generation can help in predicting what the trends may be for future generations of older adults. For example, in an analysis of nationally representative data among three generations – Baby Boomers (born 1946 to 1964), Generation X (born 1965 to 1980), and Millennials (born 1981 to 1996) – Yang and colleagues (2018) found that between 2007 and 2016, binge alcohol use and cocaine use was highest among Millennials and lowest among Baby Boomers, with Generation X somewhere in between. However, the use of crack cocaine was highest in Generation X, with prevalence rates almost twice as high compared with both Baby Boomers and Millennials. Generation X was also more likely to report use of multiple substances (excluding alcohol) compared with Millennials. It is unclear if these substance use patterns will persist as each generation ages into older adulthood, particularly since Yang and colleagues (2018) found that there was a general decline in substance use with increasing age. Nonetheless, these data suggest that Generation X, typically defined as those born between 1965 and 1980, may bring different areas of concern to practitioners with regards to substance use when they reach older adulthood, and that practitioners may need to regularly assess for other substances besides alcohol and cannabis.

Since alcohol is the most commonly used and most problematic substance among older adults, it can be helpful to know what is considered "normative" drinking for older adults. Chan and colleagues (2007) found that, among a national sample of men aged 65 and older, 29 % had zero drinks per week in the past week, 32% had one drink per week, 8% had two to three drinks per week, and 31% had more than five drinks per week. A similar pattern was observed for older women: 41% had zero drinks per week, 40% had one drink per week, 6% had two to three drinks per week, and 13% had more than two or three drinks per week. Understanding normative drinking among older adults can help practitioners compare the drinking levels of older adult clients versus these normative levels. As noted in Chapter 6, practitioners can also provide feedback to older adult clients about normative drinking levels as part of a brief intervention.

The results of the Chan and colleagues (2007) study suggest that a minority of older adults are engaging in unhealthy alcohol use. However, longitudinal data suggest that rates of unhealthy alcohol use and AUDs have increased among older adults in recent years (Breslow et al., 2017; Han et al., 2017). Han and colleagues (2017) found that participants between the ages of 50 and 64 had a 23% relative increase in past-month binge alcohol use (defined as five or more drinks on one occasion) between the years of 2005 and 2014. Adults aged 65 and older had an 11% relative increase during the same time frame. Women reported a 44% increase in past-month binge alcohol use, compared with a 9% relative increase among men, and had an 85% increase in past-month AUDs, compared with a 2% relative increase among men. Breslow and colleagues (2017) also noted increasing rates of alcohol use among adults aged 60 and over between 2007 and 2014. Specifically, the prevalence of current drinking, defined as more than one drink in the past year, increased 1% per year for men and 2% per year for women. Binge drinking, defined as five or more drinks in the same day, was stable among men but increased an average of 4% each year for women. The results of these large, national survey studies suggest that there are steady increases in drinking among older adults, and that this trend is particularly pronounced among older women. The authors noted older women's increasing use of alcohol as an emerging public health concern and encouraged regular screening in this group. Chapter 8 provides more information on unhealthy alcohol use among older women.

2.2.1 Prevalence of Unhealthy Alcohol Use Among Racial and Ethnic Minority Older Adults

White and Latinx older adults are at higher risk of unhealthy alcohol use compared with older adults from other racial/ethnic backgrounds (Assari et al., 2016; Assari et al., 2019; Han et al., 2017; Rao et al., 2015). For example, Han and colleagues (2017) found that binge alcohol use in the past month (five or more drinks on one occasion) increased significantly between 2005 and 2014 among White participants but not among participants who identified as Black, Latinx, or Asian. At the final follow-up point in 2014, Latinx participants reported the highest rate of unhealthy alcohol use in the past month (17% of participants) compared with non-Hispanic White participants. White participants also had a significant increase in past-year AUD diagnosis, defined as meeting DSM-IV criteria for either alcohol abuse or alcohol dependence, whereas no significant changes were reported for participants who identified as Black, Latinx, or Asian. In multivariate models, Asian participants were significantly less likely than White participants to endorse unhealthy alcohol use in the past month and self-reported past-year AUDs. Latinx participants were more likely to report unhealthy alcohol use in the past month compared with White participants.

Black older adults tend to drink at lower levels than other racial/ethnicity groups. In a study of Black adults 65 or older living in the Los Angeles area, 70% reported that they currently did not drink alcohol (Assari et al., 2019). In this sample, drinking alcohol was associated with financial difficulties in multivariate models controlling for other demographic and health variables. In a separate study of Black and White older adults who were part of the Religion, Aging, and Health Survey, Black and White participants had similar levels of unhealthy alcohol use (five or more drinks in a day), at around 1% of the sample. White participants were more likely to report any alcohol consumption in the past month compared with Black participants (27% vs. 15%; Assari et al., 2016).

2.2.2 International Studies on Prevalence of Unhealthy Alcohol Use Among Older Adults

A small number of international studies have examined unhealthy alcohol use among older adults. Results from the Australian National Health Survey of adults ages 55 and older indicated that abstinence from alcohol increases with age (Australian Bureau of Statistics, 2009). Alcohol consumption among women remained stable as respondents aged, whereas alcohol consumption among men decreased as respondents aged, highlighting the need to screen and assess older women who may not decrease their alcohol use with increasing age. In this survey, excessive drinking was defined as more than 168 g of alcohol per week for men and more than 112 g per week for women. This roughly translates to more than 12 standard drinks per week for men and eight standard drinks for women (there are 14 g of alcohol in a standard drink; see Section 2.1 Common Terms to Describe Alcohol Use, for more discussion on measuring standard drinks).

Rao and colleagues (2015) found that, among adults 65 and older living in the UK who were part of a large primary care dataset (Lambeth DataNet), 33% consumed alcohol in the past week, and 7% drank above recommended limits, defined as more than 21 standard drinks in a week for men and 14 for women. Lower alcohol consumption was found among participants of Asian ethnicity, Black Caribbean, and Black African ethnicity. Among participants drinking above recommended limits in the UK, the three strongest predictors were identifying as male, younger, and Irish ethnicity.

As part of the Korean Longitudinal Study of Aging of adults aged 55 and older, excessive drinking, defined as more than 14 standard drinks per week, was reported by 20% of men aged 55 to 64, 18% of men aged 65 to 74, and 11% of men aged 75 to 83. This is compared with the rates for women across the same age groups, of 0.3%, 0.6%, and 0%, respectively (French et al., 2014). In a review of drinking among older adults across different countries, Gell and colleagues (2015) concluded that rates of abstinence from alcohol among adults aged 55 and older are lowest in England and Finland and highest in the US and Korea.

2.2.3 Prevalence of Unhealthy Alcohol Use Among Sexual and Gender Minority Older Adults

There is limited research on unhealthy alcohol use among sexual and gender minority older adults. Using data from the National Survey on Drug Use and Health, Han and colleagues (2020) examined past-year alcohol and drug use among adults aged 50 and older identifying as lesbian, gay, or bisexual (LGB), as compared with heterosexual adults aged 50 and older. LGB older adults had significantly higher alcohol use (70% vs. 53%) and significantly higher rates of AUD (5% vs. 3%), as compared with heterosexual older adults. Of note, use of all other drugs except nicotine was also significantly higher among LGB older adults compared with heterosexual older adults, including cannabis, cocaine, methamphetamine, prescription opioid misuse, prescription sedative misuse, prescription tranquilizer misuse, and prescription stimulant misuse.

2.2.4 Prevalence Conclusions

For practitioners working with older adults, these studies are helpful in understanding general prevalence of unhealthy alcohol use among minority groups in the US and internationally. For racial and ethnic minority older adults, additional considerations include individual circumstances such as socioeconomic status (e.g., education and income), which are correlated yet separate from race/ethnicity. Further considerations include acculturation, which impacts drinking patterns of individuals from Latin American and Asian countries of origin (Park et al., 2014). For sexual and gender minority adults, additional considerations include the historical and current experience of anti-LGBT stigma and discrimination, as well as identity concealment and limited access to health care (Goldhammer et al., 2019). As discussed further in Chapter 8, the effects of race/ethnicity and sexual and gender minority status are important to consider in the context of screening and treatment of older adults for unhealthy alcohol use.

2.3 Comorbid Nicotine and Other Drug Use

Among those with unhealthy alcohol use, use of multiple substances (termed *polysubstance use*) is common, and practitioners should anticipate this during their interview and assessment (Crummy et al., 2020). Although research is limited about specific polysubstance use patterns among older adults, Choi and colleagues (2016) found that, among adults 50 and older who reported past-year cannabis use, 48 % had a tobacco/nicotine use disorder, 29 % had an AUD, and 8 % had other drug use disorders. Choi and DiNitto (2019) found that, among cannabis users aged 55 and older, cannabis-only admissions to ambulatory or outpatient treatment settings declined over a 5-year period, whereas admissions increased substantially for situations where cannabis was either the primary, secondary, or tertiary substance used along with other substances, highlighting the increase in polysubstance use among those seeking treatment. Among all admissions involving cannabis use, rates of concurrent unhealthy alcohol use decreased from 70 % to 62 % over the 5-year study period. Even though concurrent heroin and methamphetamine use increased, alcohol was still the primary other substance used besides cannabis, indicating that alcohol and cannabis use is a common combination among those 55 years and older. Practitioners should consider screening for both alcohol and cannabis use among older adults.

The use of cannabis among older adults has increased in recent years. This is likely because of a combination of three changes: legalization of cannabis in some countries and US states, more accepting attitudes about cannabis use (related to legalization), and Baby Boomers' increased comfort with cannabis and other psychedelic drugs compared with other generations of older adults. In the last 4 years (2015–2018) of the National Survey on Drug Use and Health, past-year cannabis use among those aged 65 and older increased from 2 % to 4 %, representing a 75 % relative increase (Han & Palamar, 2020). Rates of cannabis use for older women jumped from 2 % to

3%, representing a 93% relative increase. Practitioners may assume that older adults use cannabis for management of pain or chronic health conditions. However, Han and Palamar (2020) found that the increase in use was largely driven by older adults who had two or fewer multiple chronic medical conditions. There were also notable increases in cannabis use among older adults who regularly used alcohol in the past year.

Nicotine is also frequently used in conjunction with alcohol; in one study, 23% of those with AUD also meet criteria for a nicotine use disorder (Grant et al., 2004). Although cigarette smoking declined 28% between 2005 and 2015 among adults 18 and over, there was only a 2% decline among individuals 65 and older (Jamal et al., 2016). Henley and colleagues (2019) found that, among US adults 65 and older, 8% reported current smoking. Of those who reported smoking, White participants had the highest rates of smoking (77%), followed by Black participants (13%) and Latinx participants (7%). About half of participants (54%) who currently smoked reported a desire to quit, 47% tried to quit in the past year, and 5% successfully quit in the past year. In working with older adults with unhealthy alcohol use, practitioners should also ask about cannabis and nicotine use, assess problem severity, and consider combined approaches to reducing alcohol and other substance use.

2.4   Conclusions: Prevalence and Risk Factors

This chapter highlights several themes related to prevalence and risk factors for unhealthy alcohol use among older adults. Alcohol use exists on a continuum, with the majority of older adults drinking zero or one drink per week (Chan et al., 2007). Low-risk drinking guidelines suggested by the NIAAA can guide practitioners in understanding how to define unhealthy alcohol use, though drinking recommendations are specific to each gender and are not specific to older adults. Prevalence rates rely on the concept of a standard drink, the definition of which varies across countries. It can be useful for practitioners to educate clients on the definition of a standard drink as part of providing feedback about the client's current drinking level, discussed more in Chapter 6 on brief interventions. The prevalence data presented in this chapter indicate that the rates of unhealthy alcohol use are increasing among older adults, and there are particular concerns about unhealthy alcohol use among older women and sexual and gender minority older adults.

3

Conceptualizing Unhealthy Alcohol Use Among Older Adults

This chapter explores different ways in which practitioners might conceptualize unhealthy alcohol use among older adults. This involves consideration of ways in which processing of alcohol changes with age, as well as the age of onset of the problem (early and middle adulthood vs. older adulthood) and life transitions. The chapter also considers theoretical models of substance use (e.g., biopsychosocial model, cognitive behavioral model) and how these models apply to older adults.

3.1   Age-Related Changes in Alcohol Processing

Older adults process alcohol differently because of physiological changes that are a typical part of the aging process (Ferreira & Weems, 2008). Owing to these physiological changes, tolerance for alcohol decreases with age. This means that older adults experience the effects of alcohol more quickly at lower quantities than when they were younger. Although an older person may say that they can "hold their liquor," or that they have been "drinking the same amount for years," older adults experience increased sensitivity to alcohol and therefore their tolerance is lower than it was in their younger years.

> **Clinical Pearl**
>
> Older adults often report that the amount that they drink has not changed. This may lead a practitioner to conclude that any current problems (e.g., health or interpersonal difficulties) are not related to alcohol use. Because of the effects of sensitization, tolerance is now much lower, and the same amount of alcohol consumed when they were younger can have a potentially greater effect on medical conditions, fall risk, and cognitive status.

The following physiological changes impact older adults' ability to process alcohol, thereby increasing their sensitivity to alcohol and decreasing their tolerance:

- Decrease in muscle mass and subsequent reduction in total body water: When alcohol is consumed and processed, it is absorbed more quickly into muscle tissue than fat. With age, there is an overall decrease in muscle and an increase in fat. Over the course of adulthood, the amount of water in the body decreases by about 15% owing to a decrease in muscle mass (Malczyk et al., 2016). This means that alcohol remains in the bloodstream longer and the lengthier absorption time can also lead to higher BAC levels and increased effects, even when the person is consuming the same amount of alcohol as they did when they were younger. This decrease in total body water increases vulnerability to dehydration. Since alcohol is a diuretic, it raises further concerns about dehydration as well as contributing to lower tolerance and greater sensitivity to intoxication.
- Longer time to digest alcohol: With age, the enzyme that metabolizes alcohol (gastric alcohol dehydrogenase) decreases (Parlesak et al., 2002). This change slows absorption, leading to a higher BAC and placing greater strain on the liver since fewer enzymes are available in the stomach to assist with processing alcohol.

Although this information is specific to alcohol consumption, age-associated physiological changes can also make older adults more sensitive to alcohol–medication interactions as well as to the effects of cannabis, benzodiazepines, and opioids (Breslow et al., 2015). This will be discussed further in Chapter 4 on common comorbid conditions. Use of these substances in combination with alcohol can significantly increase the risk of falls, cognitive impairment, and other serious health problems.

3.2 Early Versus Late Onset

When conceptualizing unhealthy alcohol use among older adults, consider whether unhealthy alcohol use is new or is the continuation of a behavior established in young adulthood. Existing research on early- vs. late-onset alcohol use defines these categories: *early onset* (less than 25 years old), *late onset* (between 25 and 44 years old), and *very late onset* (over age 45; Kist et al., 2014; Wetterling et al., 2003). Unhealthy alcohol use that starts in young adulthood tends to occur daily or almost daily and continues into later life, accompanied by consequences associated with use often across multiple domains of functioning. Unhealthy alcohol use that starts in older adulthood sometimes occurs in connection with stressful life events such as retirement, loss, or the onset of a new medical problem. Questions that practitioners might ask about the course of drinking are listed in Box 1.

Box 1. Possible questions about the course of drinking

1. At what age did you start drinking on a regular basis?
2. When did you notice changes or problems with alcohol?
3. Were there periods of time in adulthood when you were not drinking? Why did you stop drinking? How long did those periods last?
4. Have changes in your drinking coincided with specific events (e.g., starting or ending a relationship; employment transitions such as retirement)?

Overall, these questions help to understand triggers and patterns of unhealthy alcohol use over time. In a qualitative study of unhealthy alcohol use among Danish adults whose unhealthy alcohol use began after age 60, Emiliussen and colleagues (2017) found three common patterns among older adults:

- Older adults with unhealthy alcohol use in younger adulthood that was not detected until older adulthood. This represents early-onset use without receiving a diagnosis until older adulthood.
- Older adults who engaged in low-risk drinking when they were younger and increased their use to an unhealthy level or developed an AUD as they got older. This represents late-onset use.
- Older adults who either did not use alcohol earlier in life or had low-risk use, which continued into older adulthood.

Research into the early- versus late-onset distinction is limited. In terms of presenting symptoms, Kist and colleagues (2014) found that scores on cognitive tests related to executive functioning, attention, and short-term memory were in the low average range for all groups, including early onset unhealthy alcohol use (younger than age 25), late onset (25–44), and very late onset (45 and older), as compared with a healthy norm group of older adults. The results did not vary by age of initiation of unhealthy alcohol use, although the authors hypothesized that the early-onset group would have worse cognitive performance compared with the other two groups. Older women tend to be disproportionately represented in those with late-onset unhealthy alcohol use (Breslow et al., 2017), whereas older men are more likely to be in the early-onset category.

In a study of adults admitted to an inpatient detoxification unit, Wetterling and colleagues (2003) found that individuals in an early-onset group (aged 25 or younger) were more likely to meet criteria for a nicotine use disorder compared with the other two groups (onset between ages 25–44 and onset after age 45), were more likely to have alcohol-related psychosocial problems (i.e., job or relationships problems because of alcohol use), were less likely to report continuous abstinence 6- and 12-months postdetoxification, and were more likely to report binge drinking. These results suggest that late-onset unhealthy alcohol use may be less severe, though still may have consequences on cognitive functioning. For older adults with less severe alcohol use, practitioners might not consider the possibility of recently developed unhealthy alcohol use because the client may be functioning fairly well.

Older adults who had a pattern of unhealthy alcohol use earlier in life are potentially at greater risk for reemergence of unhealthy alcohol use. For example, one study found that having drinking problems prior to age 50 was associated with a higher likelihood of unhealthy alcohol use later in life (Moos et al., 2010). In contrast, prior attempts to cut down on drinking and having attended Alcoholics Anonymous (AA) in the past were associated with a lower likelihood of risky drinking and alcohol-related problems in later life. This suggests that treatment experiences earlier in life may have a preventive impact on the course of unhealthy alcohol use in later life.

> **Clinical Pearl**
>
> Asking about patterns of alcohol use across the lifespan and any prior treatment can be helpful in determining whether a client has longstanding unhealthy alcohol use or if it developed more recently. That might include a question such as "how does your current level of drinking compare with that when you were in your (20s, 30s, etc.)?"

3.3   Life Transitions and Unhealthy Alcohol Use

Life transitions commonly experienced by older adults are important in the conceptualization of unhealthy alcohol use among older adults. These events may serve as triggers for increasing alcohol use. Relevant life transitions may include a change in social roles, such as retirement, adult children leaving the home, taking on a caregiving role, loss of a partner or other friends or family members, and change in functioning because of medical conditions or other situations (Satre et al., 2012). Older adults may reduce their alcohol consumption because of accumulating health effects or concerns about drinking in combination with medications. Additionally, older adults with serious chronic medical conditions such as heart problems and diabetes as well as worse overall health are more likely than others to report having stopped drinking altogether (Satre et al., 2007).

Unhealthy alcohol use tends to shift in predictable ways across the adult lifespan, with an overall decrease in use coinciding with the onset of new social roles in younger adulthood such as parenthood and employment (Leggat et al., 2021). In older adults, increases in drinking may occur as social roles shift toward retirement, and older adults no longer have the same responsibilities that came with employment or parenting (Kuerbis & Sacco, 2012). Older adults may drink more to cope with the changes that come with these life transitions. As with younger adults, loss of a partner through separation, divorce, or death can lead to increased drinking among older adults (Satre et al., 2012).

It can be valuable for practitioners to explore lifespan patterns of alcohol use with older adult clients, and to consider what events may have triggered increases in alcohol use to an unhealthy level. For example, a nationally representative study of alcohol use patterns among adults in New Zealand found that drinking patterns were largely stable across adulthood, with the norm within individuals being either long periods of low-risk alcohol use or long periods of unhealthy use. The transition from low-risk use to unhealthy use was uncommon and was related to unemployment, relationship problems, and chronic health problems (Towers et al., 2018). This suggests that there are a few possible patterns of unhealthy alcohol use among older adults. First, older adults may have engaged in low-risk drinking for much of their adult life, at which point a life transition such as retirement or loss leads them to consume unhealthy amounts of alcohol. A second possible pattern occurs when older adults have been drinking at unhealthy levels throughout much of their life. This pattern may include chronic unhealthy alcohol use or intermittent unhealthy alcohol use in response to life stressors during adulthood and aging. Finally, older adults who have been abstinent for many years may start drinking again, consistent with a pattern of returning to drinking. Regardless of the specific pattern of alcohol use, an assessment of how life events influenced alcohol use can aid practitioners in conceptualizing the role of alcohol in an older adult's life.

3.4 Biopsychosocial Model

Unhealthy alcohol use among older adults can be informed by the *biopsychosocial model*, which is frequently used in the aging literature and in the health psychology literature (Lehman et al., 2017). The biopsychosocial model considers multiple influences on the development of mental health or behavioral problems such as unhealthy alcohol use (Highland et al., 2013) – that is, unhealthy alcohol use is not considered solely related to functioning in one domain but rather the interaction of multiple domains, including genetics, sociocultural influences, and psychological factors (Skewes & Gonzalez, 2013). Applied to older adults, relevant biological components may include genetic risk, the presence of chronic medical conditions, chronic pain, and the normative changes in physiology causing increased sensitivity to alcohol and decreased tolerance. Examples of psychological factors particularly relevant to older adults include mental health conditions such as anxiety and depression, social skills, beliefs and expectations around alcohol use, and personality traits such as extroversion. Social influences include any recent life transitions that lead to loss of social support, such as retirement or loss of a spouse or partner, alcohol use norms among partners and family, peer relationships, or intimate relationships, cultural beliefs around alcohol use, and socioeconomic status.

When working with older adults, it is useful to think about how the various components of the biopsychosocial model have changed for the older client across adulthood. For example, family relationships (e.g., shifting family dynamics, loss of a partner to death or divorce) and psychological well-being (e.g., increases in stress) have likely changed over the course of an older adult's life, and exploring these issues with clients can be helpful to understanding factors that may have contributed to unhealthy alcohol use. Components of the biopsychosocial model interact with each other over time. In this way, a biological factor (e.g., decreased mobility or other medical problems) may influence the older person's ability to spend time with trusted friends (a social factor), thereby increasing the likelihood that alcohol may be used to combat loneliness. Using the biopsychosocial model for conceptualizing unhealthy alcohol use among older adults allows practitioners to see a broader picture of contextual variables that are related to alcohol use. Figure 1 provides an example of how components of the biopsychosocial model may interact for older adults with unhealthy alcohol use.

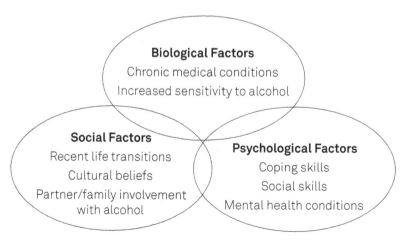

Figure 1.   Biopsychosocial model for unhealthy alcohol use among older adults.

3.5 Stress and Coping Framework

Stress and coping models propose that unhealthy alcohol use is one way in which individuals respond to stressful life circumstances, including problems with friends and family members, work, finances, and other situations (Moos, 2007). The experience of these problems may lead to distress and further isolation, increasing the chances of unhealthy alcohol use. The ways in which individuals respond to stress may be reflected in their coping style. Coping styles are typically delineated into problem- or emotion-focused coping and are also characterized by approach- or avoidance-based strategies. Examples of problem-focused and approach-based coping include efforts to change or modify a difficult situation, whereas examples of emotion-focused and avoidance-based coping include efforts such as engaging in activities to manage emotions. Approach coping is characterized by strategies such as problem solving, seeking support or guidance, or engaging in positive reappraisal. In contrast, avoidance coping is characterized by avoiding direct communication with others, venting one's feelings (especially anger) onto others, and/or engaging in unsafe health behaviors to reduce tension (e.g., unhealthy alcohol use). Although almost everyone uses both strategies at times, and there are aspects of each strategy that can be adaptive, emotion-focused and avoidance-based coping is considered less adaptive than problem-focused and approach-based coping, and tends to be associated with unsatisfactory outcomes.

Evidence suggests that there are age-related differences in coping strategies. Older adults tend to engage in less avoidance coping and similar or higher levels of approach coping compared with other age groups (Amirkhan & Auyeung, 2007). In light of this, practitioners may notice that older adults can be more effective at employing adaptive coping strategies than younger adults. There is some support, however, for the idea that all types of coping decrease with age, especially among adults over the age of 80 (Brennan et al., 2012). This may reflect an effort to anticipate stressors before they happen. Owing to these potential age-related differences/improvements in coping, practitioners may be less likely to see older adults engaging in alcohol use for coping motives compared with their younger clients, due in part to their greater experience managing difficult situations throughout life.

In support of stress and coping theories of unhealthy alcohol use, researchers have investigated specific challenges associated with aging (e.g., pain, disability, death of family members) as risk factors in the development or exacerbation of unhealthy alcohol use. Research studies examining stressful events and drinking are correlational, though they demonstrate a relationship between such events and increased drinking. For instance, one study found that individuals who used drinking to cope with stress were more likely to engage in unhealthy alcohol use over a 20-year period (Moos et al., 2010). Additionally, in a nationally representative sample of adults aged 60 and older, Sacco and colleagues (2014) found that stressful life events were associated with past-year AUD diagnosis, and that higher perceived stress was associated with past-year AUD diagnosis among older men. Among older women in the sample, high levels of perceived stress were associated with lower daily alcohol consumption. In a nationwide sample of adults aged 65 and over, Shaw and colleagues (2011) found a direct relationship between higher levels of financial strain and unhealthy alcohol use among older men. These findings indicate that, at least for some older adults, stressors and negative events that occur more frequently in later life are associated with unhealthy alcohol use.

As in other age groups, the use of alcohol for coping with negative emotions may occur among older adults with a history of trauma, including symptoms of posttraumatic stress disorder (PTSD). Older adults may be reluctant to disclose past experiences of trauma, although they can benefit substantially from evidence-based behavioral treatments for trauma, including exposure-based interventions (Cook et al., 2017). The association between early trauma in childhood and health problems in later life, including unhealthy alcohol use and other substance use, is well-established (Goodman, 2017). Therefore, practitioners may need to assess and treat traumatic experiences among older adults, which may in turn reduce the use of alcohol for coping with PTSD symptoms, anxiety, and other negative emotions. This is referred to as *trauma-informed care*, and it can be integrated into existing substance use treatments.

Clinical Pearl

Older adults may not want to revisit traumas that happened in their childhood or young adulthood, reporting to practitioners that they have already dealt with events in the distant past. As an example, an older client with a long history of trauma, drug, and alcohol use told their practitioner, "They always want to talk about my childhood, and I'm done talking about that." This requires sensitivity on the part of the practitioner and a respect for the client's autonomy in deciding what to discuss during treatment. However, older adults can benefit from evidence-based interventions that address co-occurring unhealthy alcohol use and PTSD.

3.6 Cognitive Behavioral Model

Broadly, the *cognitive behavioral model* frames alcohol use in the context of antecedents and consequences, while also examining the ways in which thoughts serve to maintain alcohol use (Higgins et al., 2021). Identification of antecedents allows clients to increase awareness of high-risk situations and either try to avoid those situations or use coping skills to manage situations. Identification of antecedents can also help the client discover patterns of behavior that increase the likelihood of alcohol use – for example, specific individuals, places, or situations. In the cognitive behavioral model, thoughts may serve to reinforce and maintain alcohol use – for example, when a client drinks in response to a craving for alcohol and thinks "it isn't worth trying to reduce my drinking. I am never going to succeed at cutting back."

Antecedents, sometimes called triggers, occur prior to drinking and increase the likelihood that alcohol use will occur. Antecedents involve social, behavioral, cognitive, or physiological factors that are associated with drinking (see Table 3). Social antecedents include being around certain individuals, pressure to drink from others (or the general tendency to act the way that others are acting), and the stress associated with interpersonal conflict. Behavioral antecedents include environmental triggers, such as particular places (restaurants, bars, etc.), being with others who also drink, or attending events that serve alcohol. Cognitive antecedents include specific emotions that trigger drinking (anger, depression), or underlying beliefs that alcohol use is helpful in managing stress or in having more fun. Common emotions that trigger drinking among older adults are depression, boredom, and loneliness (Schonfeld, 2020). Expectancies are another category of beliefs associated with alcohol use behavior. For example, the idea that "Once I have a few drinks I'm going to feel more relaxed" is a typical positive expectancy of what might happen when alcohol is consumed. Physiological triggers include drinking in response to medical conditions (e.g., sleep problems or chronic pain) or drinking in response to withdrawal symptoms.

Older adults may have additional antecedents, including coping with chronic medical problems, more difficulty scheduling pleasant events because of mobility and transportation issues, loneliness, or social pressure associated with living in retirement communities in which drinking offers a means of interacting with others (Immonen et al., 2010). Generally, having multiple kinds of reinforcing activities, from hobbies to meaningful social relationships, decreases the likelihood of unhealthy alcohol use (Andrabi et al., 2017). For some older adults, retirement leads to fewer opportunities for social interaction and meaningful activity. Retirement may include negative aspects such as loss of status or of supportive social rela-

Table 3. Antecedents and consequences of drinking in the cognitive behavioral model

Examples of antecedents	Examples of consequences
Social antecedents: Pressure to drink from friends and/or family, conflict with friends and/or family, or lack of reinforcing activities, potentially linked to retirement.	Social consequences: In the short-term, reinforcement or praise from friends and/or family. In the long-term, may create tension in social relationships.
Behavioral antecedents: Specific locations or situations associated with drinking, such as after dinner or with a specific group of friends.	Behavioral consequences: These locations or situations can serve as a reminder or trigger for drinking.
Cognitive antecedents: Negative thoughts about oneself, or negative mood states such as anger, depression, or loneliness.	Cognitive consequences: In the short-term, increase in positive thoughts and emotions and reduction in negative thoughts and emotions. In the long-term, negative thoughts about oneself may increase.
Physiological antecedents: Sleep problems, chronic pain, or management of other chronic medical conditions.	Physiological consequences: May feel better physically in the short-term, though conditions may worsen over the long-term with continued alcohol use.

tionships at work and professional identity, or positive aspects such as increased leisure time. In a qualitative study of 12 Danish older adults with onset of AUDs after age 60, interview participants described retirement-related changes during this period of life as "being somebody and becoming nobody" (Emiliussen et al., 2017, p. 978). Interviewees also reported a lack of meaningful activity and the use of retirement as a reason to engage in celebratory drinking, which then led to unhealthy alcohol use.

In addition to considering the antecedents of alcohol use, the cognitive behavioral model proposes that consequences of use can serve to reinforce ongoing use or to motivate cutting back (see Table 3). Consequences fall into different categories, including social, cognitive, and physiological. For example, positive social consequences can include the enjoyment that comes from being with friends when drinking; negative social consequences might include experiencing embarrassment or disapproval from others. Cognitive and emotional consequences can include increased positive thoughts or reduction in unpleasant emotions such as anxiety and depression. Positive physiological consequences may include temporary reduction in pain; negative physiological consequences include the unpleasant feelings that come with a hangover as well as more serious health problems (e.g., an injury because of falling or liver damage that develops as a result of chronic drinking). As will be further described in Chapter 6, understanding these cognitive and behavioral factors and the role they play in alcohol use informs a number of key intervention strategies.

3.7 Conclusions: Conceptualizing Unhealthy Alcohol Use

Unhealthy alcohol use among older adults can be understood from multiple perspectives, a summary of which is provided in Table 4. Many of these perspectives need to be considered when a practitioner is trying to understand what maintains unhealthy alcohol use. First, alcohol processing changes with age, making older adults more susceptible to the effects of alcohol. The age of onset of the problems helps practitioners determine the pattern of alcohol use and whether it is a new or long-standing problem. Patterns of alcohol use may be influenced by recent life transitions, coping styles, and recent stressors, as well as factors that fall within the biopsychosocial model. Finally, a cognitive behavioral framework can assist in understanding the proximal antecedents and consequences that maintain unhealthy alcohol use.

Table 4. Conceptualizing older adult unhealthy alcohol use

Age-related changes in alcohol processing	Increased sensitivity to alcohol means that problems may emerge at lower levels of alcohol use.
Age of onset	Understand the lifespan pattern of alcohol use, including whether unhealthy alcohol use started in younger adulthood or in later life.
Life transitions	Life transitions such as loss and retirement can increase risk for developing unhealthy alcohol use.
Biopsychosocial model	Physiological factors (lower tolerance, increased sensitivity), psychological factors (coping and mental health problems), and social factors (life transitions, partner drinking) contribute to unhealthy alcohol use.
Stress and coping framework	Stressful events, trauma, and avoidant behavior patterns may lead to unhealthy alcohol use.
Cognitive behavioral model	Unhealthy alcohol use can be understood in the context of antecedents and consequences.

4

Diagnosing Unhealthy Alcohol Use Among Older Adults

This chapter reviews the *Diagnostic and Statistical Manual of Mental Disorders,* 5th edition (DSM-5) criteria for alcohol use disorder (AUD) as well as ways in which the criteria may miss many older adults with unhealthy alcohol use. Common signs of unhealthy alcohol use are discussed, as well as differential diagnosis and common conditions that are comorbid with AUD and unhealthy alcohol use.

4.1   DSM-5 Criteria for Alcohol Use Disorder

The DSM-5 defines substance use disorders (including AUDs) according to 11 diagnostic criteria (American Psychiatric Association, 2013). To meet criteria for a *mild* specifier, two to three symptoms need to be present; for a *moderate* specifier, four to five symptoms, and for *severe*, six or more symptoms need to be present. Below is a subset of diagnostic criteria for AUD along with a discussion of how these criteria may be problematic for older adults. Specifically, there is a concern that the DSM-5 criteria may miss older adults with unhealthy alcohol use, resulting in underdiagnosis (Kuerbis, 2020).

- **Larger amounts of alcohol are taken, or alcohol is consumed over a longer period of time, than planned:** Because of age-related cognitive changes or mild cognitive impairment, some older adults may have difficulty monitoring how much they consume and determining whether that represents increases in the intended amount or duration. Therefore, self-reported alcohol quantity may have limited diagnostic value.

> **Clinical Pearl**
>
> For older adults, an AUD diagnosis based on the criterion of increasing amounts of alcohol consumed over time may lead to underdiagnosis. Remember that the sensitization process means that the same amount of alcohol consumed in older adulthood may now cause problems that were not present in younger adulthood. Rather, look for unsuccessful efforts to cut back, withdrawal, and social and/or interpersonal problems, which Kuerbis (2020) found were the criteria most successful in diagnosing AUD among older adults.

- **A significant amount of time is spent trying to obtain alcohol, consume alcohol, or recover from drinking alcohol:** Older adults may take longer than younger adults to recover from the effects of small amounts of alcohol (related to reduced tolerance, as discussed in Section 3.1 Age-Related Changes in Alcohol Processing). This means that the amount of time spent recovering may indicate reduction in tolerance rather than substantial alcohol use.
- **Alcohol use results in a failure to fulfill roles, such as at work, school, or home:** The social and occupational roles that older adults have may not match the obligations usually associated with this criterion (e.g., work, school, or home). Therefore, practitioners may need to think broadly about older clients' current responsibilities and activities (e.g., helping family members, volunteer commitments).

> **Clinical Pearl**
>
> Some of the roles that older adults fill include caregiving to other family members, volunteering, and/or providing child care for grandchildren. There may be others, and disengagement from any of these roles may indicate unhealthy alcohol use.

- **Alcohol use continues despite ongoing social and/or interpersonal problems caused or made worse by alcohol:** There are two aspects of this criterion that are problematic with older adults. First, older adults may not attribute the problems they experience to alcohol use, especially if their drinking levels have not increased. Compounding this problem, practitioners may inaccurately attribute "ongoing social or interpersonal problems" to typical aging or to other medical conditions and may neglect to consider that these problems are alcohol-related.
- **Alcohol is used in situations in which its use is physically hazardous:** Older adults may be less likely to engage in potentially hazardous activities, particularly if they do not drive regularly.
- **Tolerance, marked by the need for increasing amounts of alcohol or diminished effect of alcohol while consuming the same amount:** Older adults generally have lower tolerance for alcohol owing to the increased sensitivity described previously (see Section 3.1). This goes against the typical pattern of increased tolerance with greater use over time, and may cause a practitioner to evaluate this criterion incorrectly.
- **Withdrawal, marked by alcohol withdrawal symptoms or by taking another substance to manage alcohol withdrawal symptoms:** Some older adults have "late-onset" unhealthy alcohol use that started or be-

came unhealthy later in life. These individuals might not develop a typical physiological dependence profile and therefore may not show classic signs of withdrawal. At the same time, older adults with nonproblematic (low-risk) alcohol use may develop physiological dependence quickly. Finally, alcohol withdrawal symptoms among older adults can be more subtle than what is typically expected by practitioners who are used to working primarily with younger clients (see Han & Moore, 2018).

In summary, there are many concerns about whether the DSM-5 criteria for AUDs adequately capture the experience of older adults with unhealthy alcohol use. Analyzing data from the 2009 National Survey on Drug Use and Health, Kuerbis and colleagues (2013) found that, among adults aged 50 and older, the DSM-5 criteria for AUD identified only severe cases of AUD in this age group, suggesting that the criteria may be less effective in detecting lower-severity problems among older adults. Because of this, practitioners may find that unhealthy alcohol use is particularly easy to miss among older adults. This leads to underdiagnosis, misdiagnosis, and undertreatment of unhealthy alcohol use in this population. When using the DSM-5, practitioners should consider the possibility that older clients who do not meet criteria for AUDs may still benefit from a clinical intervention. Interventions for unhealthy alcohol use are discussed in Chapter 6. Additionally, practitioners can focus on personal consequences of alcohol use, regardless of whether the older adult meets criteria for a DSM-5 diagnosis.

4.2   Identification of Unhealthy Alcohol Use and Diagnosis

When meeting with an older adult client, practitioners need to consider whether presenting symptoms are consistent with unhealthy alcohol use or are a sign of another physical or mental health condition. For example, symptoms of unhealthy alcohol use may include confusion or memory problems. These symptoms could also be indicative of delirium, dementia, or another underlying medical condition such as hypertension. It is important to consider the possibility of unhealthy alcohol use in a differential diagnosis, while also being aware that symptoms of unhealthy alcohol use overlap with other medical conditions that may require physician evaluation. In this section, common symptoms of unhealthy alcohol use are reviewed, as well as presenting problems that have overlapping symptoms with unhealthy alcohol use among older adults.

4.2.1 Common Signs of Unhealthy Alcohol Use

Common signs that might suggest unhealthy alcohol use include:
- Short-term memory loss
- Difficulties in judgment and decision making
- Fluctuations in weight and/or changes in appetite
- Isolation from family and friends or a change in social groups
- Lethargy/low energy
- Difficulties in work, school, or other roles
- Falls and/or bruises
- Change in personal hygiene
- Trouble adhering to prescription medications
- Changes in financial status, such as requesting to borrow money or spending more money than usual
- Changes in sleep patterns

Although this list of common signs of unhealthy alcohol use is not exhaustive, these concerns may also be signs of other mental health conditions (e.g., depression). Because of this, differential diagnosis with regard to unhealthy alcohol use among older adults can be complex, because the symptoms often overlap with symptoms of many other conditions (see Kuerbis, 2020, for a review). For example, infections, sleep problems, and chronic health conditions such as diabetes and chronic obstructive pulmonary disease can also lead to lethargy and low energy. Table 5 highlights why differential diagnosis may be complicated. Symptoms are often shared between multiple conditions common to older adults, including unhealthy alcohol use.

As can be seen in Table 5, many of the signs of unhealthy alcohol use could be overlooked and attributed to typical aging or another psychiatric or medical condition. Therefore, lack of adequate consideration of unhealthy alcohol use is a risk in differential diagnosis with older adults.

4.3 Differential Diagnoses to Consider

It is possible for symptoms of unhealthy alcohol use to resemble a number of other medical or psychiatric conditions. When in doubt, practitioners should refer clients for a medical evaluation. Below are some common clinical situations where symptoms described by older adults may overlap with symptoms of unhealthy alcohol use (see Dar 2006; Kuerbis, 2020, for a review):
- **Medical conditions:** Untreated or poorly managed chronic medical conditions can lead to similar symptoms to those of unhealthy alcohol use,

4 Diagnosing Unhealthy Alcohol Use Among Older Adults

Table 5. Symptoms shared with unhealthy alcohol use

Symptoms	Clinical implications for alcohol use
Short-term memory loss or other cognitive changes	Age-related declines in working memory and short-term memory are common among older adults. These could indicate age-related declines, depression, anxiety, or an underlying medical condition, in addition to unhealthy alcohol use.
Fluctuations in weight and/or changes in appetite	Changes in appetite and weight may occur because of side effects of some prescription medications. Excessive weight gain could also be a result of unhealthy alcohol use, while weight loss or poor nutrition may be associated with skipping meals or poor diet.
Isolation from family and friends or a change in social groups	Some older adults live alone and this is associated with increased risk of loneliness. Loneliness can be an indication of depression or might be dismissed by health care professionals as a typical part of aging. On the other hand, social isolation may be a consequence of unhealthy alcohol use, because of time spent drinking alone and resulting loss of social connections.
Lethargy or low energy	Older adults may experience fatigue owing to medical conditions, pain, or medication side effects. Practitioners might assume that a client is experiencing low energy as a typical part of aging. Lethargy can also be an indicator of unhealthy alcohol use as individuals may feel sluggish after drinking heavily or have alcohol-related sleep disruptions.
Difficulties in work, school, or other roles	The roles that older adults occupy are often different from those of adults in other life stages. Older adults who are retired often have other responsibilities, such as helping members of their family or volunteering. Problems in fulfilling these interpersonal roles can be because of a mental health condition or unhealthy alcohol use.
Falls and/or bruises	Falls can result from side effects of new medication or medication interactions, and can also be a sign of unhealthy alcohol use.
Change in personal hygiene	A change in personal hygiene can be related to change in mood, such as an increase in depression or anxiety symptoms, as well as an indicator of unhealthy alcohol use.

Table 5. continued

Symptoms	Clinical implications for alcohol use
Change in financial status, such as requesting to borrow money or spending more money than usual	Because sensitivity to alcohol is higher and tolerance is lower, older adults can develop unhealthy alcohol use without spending a significant amount of money on alcohol. This is in contrast to younger adults who might spend a larger amount of money on alcohol as their tolerance increases. However, older adults are particularly vulnerable to scams and other forms of financial abuse, and unhealthy alcohol use increases the likelihood of poor decision making.
Changes in sleep patterns	Some changes in sleep are common for older adults, including lighter sleep, more nighttime awakenings, and (consequently) more daytime napping. Alcohol use is known to make these problems worse. It can be difficult to determine whether sleep changes are associated with aging or a different condition, such as unhealthy alcohol use.

including lethargy, cognitive problems, sleep problems, and weight fluctuation.

- **Mild cognitive impairment or dementia:** Cognitive changes may also be a symptom of alcohol use, particularly memory problems and poor judgment and decision making, resulting from long-term unhealthy alcohol use.
- **Major depressive disorder and/or persistent depressive disorder:** Changes in cognitive functioning, sleep, appetite, energy, and social engagement are also symptoms of unhealthy alcohol use.
- **Anxiety disorders:** Symptoms that are common to anxiety disorders, including sleep disturbance, being easily fatigued, and difficulty concentrating may also be signs of unhealthy alcohol use.

Table 6 lists conditions that can have similar symptoms to those of unhealthy alcohol use or AUDs and how to differentiate between the conditions.

As can be seen from the information in Tables 5 and 6, differential diagnosis of unhealthy alcohol use can be complex, due to the high level of overlap of symptoms with other conditions. Symptoms need to be evaluated carefully to determine the presence of unhealthy alcohol use.

Table 6. Presenting problems appearing similar to unhealthy alcohol use

Clinical presentation	Characteristics that differ from unhealthy alcohol use
Chronic medical conditions	There can be significant overlap between symptoms of unhealthy alcohol use and chronic medical conditions among older adults. Care coordination is important to determine whether medical conditions overlap with symptoms of unhealthy alcohol use (see the section Care Coordination, in Chapter 6).
Mild cognitive impairment or dementia	Declines in cognitive status have been present for a significant amount of time, often for months or years, and abilities show a downward trend. Cognitive impairment related to alcohol use may show more fluctuation based on alcohol consumption.
Major depressive disorder (MDD); persistent depressive disorder (PDD)	MDD and/or PDD is often comorbid with unhealthy alcohol use, with significant overlap of symptoms, and can act as an antecedent to unhealthy alcohol use among older adults. The presence of a sense of worthlessness or negative self-evaluation can help differentiate MDD and/or PDD from unhealthy alcohol use. The Patient Health Questionnaire-9 (PHQ-9) is suggested for assessing depression symptoms among older adults (Kroenke et al., 2001; also see Appendix 1).
Anxiety disorders	Anxiety disorders are often comorbid with unhealthy alcohol use and alcohol may be used to manage symptoms. The presence of excessive worry can help differentiate anxiety from unhealthy alcohol use. The Generalized Anxiety Disorder Screener (GAD-7) is suggested for assessing anxiety symptoms among older adults (Wild et al., 2014; see also Appendix 2).

4.3.1 Cognitive Changes With Age

There is variability in the extent to which individuals experience cognitive changes as they age, which is relevant to the discussion of differential diagnosis (Harada et al., 2013). An older adult client may present with cognitive changes, which could be a symptom of a number of diagnoses, including unhealthy alcohol use. It is helpful for practitioners to know typical age-related changes in cognition to aid in separating the changes from symptoms of other diagnoses. Of note, the magnitude of cognitive changes for otherwise healthy older adults is modest until the 80s, and there is no noticeable decline in verbal ability until the late 80s (Schaie, 1994). Speed of processing, which has to do with how quickly cognitive tasks are performed, declines with age, typically starting to slow down in one's 30s and continuing to slow throughout one's life (Salthouse, 2010). Older adults show declines in working memory, or the ability to hold chunks of information in mind for a short time, compared with younger adults. There is also age-related decline in reasoning and spatial visualization, which is typically defined as the ability to mentally manipulate 2D and 3D figures (Salthouse, 2010). One's vocabulary tends to remain stable or even improve with age, in tandem with overall stability in language skills (Johnson et al., 2018).

Procedural memory, a kind of nondeclarative memory, is about how to perform motor activities like riding a bike or tying one's shoes. These abilities tend to stay intact with age and therefore remain relatively unchanged. Declarative memory includes episodic memory (memory for events) and semantic memory (general knowledge). Episodic memory, particularly memory for recent events such as those occurring in the past week, tends to decline the most starting in middle age.

Executive functioning generally includes higher-order thought processes such as planning ahead, solving novel problems, organizing information, and flexibly switching from one task to another. Aging has variable effects on executive functioning abilities. Concept formation, the ability to inhibit responses, and mental flexibility decline with age, especially after age 70, whereas other skills, such as the ability to find similarities between things, tends to remain stable (Harada et al., 2013).

In summary, many older adults will experience declines in cognition that are considered typical for their age. At the same time, practitioners should be aware that problems around cognition for older adults could signal consequences of unhealthy alcohol use or other diagnoses. Practitioners can take a thorough history to understand the nature of the cognitive changes and whether the changes coincide with any other health behaviors, such as unhealthy alcohol use. If cognitive changes are beyond what is expected for the person's age, and other conditions such as unhealthy alcohol use have been ruled out, practitioners might consider a referral to a neuropsychologist to better assess cognitive processes.

4.3.2 Long-Term Alcohol Use and Cognitive Impairment

Korsakoff's syndrome is a type of dementia that can result from long-term, unhealthy alcohol use and thiamine deficiency, though it can also result from other medical conditions (Isenberg-Grzeda et al., 2012). Occasionally it can be reversed if detected very early. Older adults with memory loss or other dementia symptoms who report a history of substantial alcohol use may benefit from neuropsychological testing. In the absence of continued alcohol use, deficits resulting from Korsakoff's syndrome tend to be static, whereas cognitive impairment associated with Alzheimer's disease continues to increase over time. Among older adults who have stopped drinking, the static nature of Korsakoff's syndrome is characterized by deficits that do not improve but also do not decline further. There are other ways in which unhealthy alcohol use can lead to brain damage and cognitive decline, such as through alcohol-related high blood pressure, cerebrovascular disease, and subsequent vascular dementia.

4.4   Comorbid Medical and Mental Health Conditions

Although full consideration of medical conditions that may co-occur with unhealthy alcohol use is beyond the scope of this book, below are some of the most common comorbid medical conditions. Alcohol use can worsen many of these problems. Additionally, these medical conditions may be treated with prescription medications that have an adverse impact when combined with alcohol. Common medications that negatively interact with alcohol among older adults include aspirin, acetaminophen, cold and allergy medicine (antihistamines), cough syrup, sleeping medication, pain medication, anxiolytics, antihypertensives, and antidepressants (NIAAA, 2014). Table 7 describes common comorbid medical conditions among older adults with unhealthy alcohol use, including key ways in which these conditions are impacted by use of alcohol.

4.4.1   Comorbid Mental Health Conditions

It is common for older adult clients presenting with unhealthy alcohol use to also have other mental health conditions. For example, in a national sample of Medicare beneficiaries aged 65 and older, 24 % of those with a past-year substance use disorder diagnosis received treatment in the past year for a mental health condition, compared with 12 % of those without a substance use disorder diagnosis (Parish et al., 2022). Those with a substance use disorder diagnosis were also more likely to report past-year serious psychological distress (14 % vs. 4 %) and past-year suicidal ideation (7 % vs. 2 %) as compared to those without a substance use disorder diagnosis. Practitioners should be mindful that clients may use alcohol to cope with symptoms of depression and anxiety, and additionally, these symptoms may also be a consequence of drinking. Depression and anxiety symptoms may have a negative effect on substance use treatment outcomes (Wolitzky-Taylor et al., 2015).

Table 7. Common comorbid medical conditions

Condition	Impact of alcohol on condition
Type 2 diabetes	Alcohol damages the pancreas and can also stop the liver from breaking down sugars, leading to higher blood glucose levels.
Decreased bone density (osteoporosis)	Unhealthy alcohol use can affect the body's calcium levels and lead to bone density problems.
Depression, anxiety, and other mental health disorders	Mood disorders may lead to the use of alcohol for coping. Conversely, preexisting unhealthy alcohol use increases the likelihood of developing mood disorders due, in part, to the reduction in other previously enjoyable activities, sleep disruption, and other consequences of unhealthy alcohol use.
Cirrhosis and other liver diseases	The liver can be significantly damaged by long-term alcohol use, resulting first in fatty liver disease and then cirrhosis.
Hypertension and other cardiovascular problems	Alcohol use over time can increase blood pressure levels, leading to hypertension, heart attacks, and strokes.
Cognitive impairment	Long-term alcohol use can lead to significant cognitive impairments later in life. Although this is sometimes a differential diagnosis question (Does the older adult with cognitive impairment actually have unhealthy alcohol use or an AUD?), the more common picture is one of comorbidity. This may limit the types of treatments in which the client can engage. Behavioral treatment options may be more appropriate than cognitive options for older adults with cognitive impairments.
Poor immune functioning	Alcohol use results in impairments in the immune system, which increases susceptibility to pneumonia and other infectious diseases. Because of this, reduction or abstinence goals may be more critical for older adults.
Cancer	Many studies show that alcohol use increases risk for cancers, including those of the mouth, throat, colon, breast, and liver.

Even for older adults who use alcohol at a level that does not meet criteria for a diagnosis, there are several reasons why alcohol use at lower levels can be problematic for mental health. For example, moderate drinking can worsen sleep, leading to fatigue, and has the potential to reduce antidepressant response and increase the risk of side effects such as drowsiness, dizziness, and increased feelings of depression or hopelessness (NIAAA, 2014). Older adults with depression are already at an elevated risk for suicide, and alcohol use is an additional risk factor, particularly during periods of intoxication. For example, Choi and colleagues (2018) found that, among older adults aged 50 and older who committed suicide, 32% had a positive blood alcohol content, and two thirds of those individuals had a BAC ≥ 0.08 g/dl, indicating intoxication at the time of death.

For these reasons, identification and treatment of unhealthy alcohol use among older adults with depression, anxiety, or other mental health problems is critical (van den Berg et al., 2014). Some individuals with alcohol and other substance use problems first seek mental health treatment or may present in a primary care or other medical settings. Motivational and cognitive behavioral interventions can be integrated into mental health care and prevent escalation of unhealthy alcohol use. Mental health symptoms often improve when those with anxiety and depression cut back on alcohol use (Bahorik et al., 2016).

4.5 Conclusions: Diagnosing Unhealthy Alcohol Use

Older adults are at risk for underdiagnosis of unhealthy alcohol use, and this may be related to the way in which the DSM-5 criteria for AUD are worded. Older adults are more likely than other age groups to be "diagnostic orphans" when it comes to AUD, meaning that they meet one of the DSM-5 criteria but fail to meet enough criteria for a diagnosis and subsequent treatment (Kuerbis, 2020). Practitioners should consider that unhealthy alcohol use can often look like other conditions among older adults, such as mood disorders, anxiety disorders, or cognitive impairment. Unhealthy alcohol use is frequently comorbid with both physical and mental health diagnoses, and can often serve to worsen the course and outcome of comorbid conditions.

5

Screening and Assessment

Medical and social services settings are now integrating routine screening for behavioral health concerns for all clients, including screening for unhealthy alcohol use. However, some individuals may still be overlooked in the screening process, including older adults (Han & Moore, 2018). Annual screening gives practitioners a greater opportunity to detect and address unhealthy alcohol use before an individual suffers severe consequences. It also normalizes conversations about unhealthy alcohol use, reducing the stigma surrounding unhealthy alcohol use and reinforcing the idea that a discussion about substance use is an important aspect of overall health. Systematic screening offers an opportunity for practitioners to inquire about recent drinking patterns and inform clients about the recommended alcohol consumption levels. It can also lead to earlier detection of unhealthy alcohol use and related problems. A positive screen can trigger a more comprehensive assessment of unhealthy alcohol use. This chapter focuses on screening recommendations, clinical interviewing, and appropriate assessment instruments for unhealthy alcohol use among older adults.

Screening older adults for alcohol use can occur across many settings. Places where older adults receive social services (e.g., senior centers, retirement communities, assisted living facilities, and long-term care facilities) provide opportunities for alcohol screening among older adults who might not routinely access medical care. Sacco and colleagues (2015) evaluated alcohol use among older adults living in a retirement community in the suburbs of Washington, DC, using the Alcohol Use Disorders Identification Test (AUDIT; see Section 5.3.1 Alcohol Use Disorders Identification Test). Over half of the retirement community residents interviewed (57 %) reported drinking on about 4 days per week, and many (43 %) reported drinking alone, most commonly in their apartments. Unhealthy alcohol use was uncommon (3 %), although 47 % were drinking above recommended guidelines, and 62 % endorsed a medication interaction risk. Schonfeld (2020) noted that social activities at retirement communities tend to revolve around drinking, further reinforcing the need to screen across multiple settings.

Non-White clients are less likely to be routinely screened for alcohol use, despite recent increases in drinking among all populations (Chen et al., 2020), but especially in racial and ethnic minority subgroups (Grant et al., 2017). Additionally, older women are emerging as a group of concern for alcohol use, and may potentially be overlooked in screening because of preconceived notions that men are more likely to have unhealthy alcohol use than women (Han et al., 2017). Recent survey data suggest that rates of unhealthy alcohol use and AUDs are increasing more rapidly among older women compared with older men (Han et al., 2017). In light of these findings, practitioners need to be mindful to screen all clients for unhealthy alcohol use.

5.1 Screening Recommendations

Current guidelines recommend yearly screening for unhealthy alcohol use among older adults in health care settings (Substance Abuse and Mental Health Services Administration [SAMHSA], 2020). Practitioners should normalize screening by saying, "I ask all my clients about their alcohol use," to help reduce stigma and minimize the chances of a client feeling singled out. To build rapport while simultaneously gaining a better understanding of a client's drinking, it can be useful to ask open-ended questions regarding the context of drinking and any problems they may have experienced in connection with alcohol use. In addition, practitioners should ask about the client's usual quantity and frequency of alcohol consumption, as well as how often they have had four or more drinks on any 1 day during the prior year (a lower threshold for binge drinking than is typically used). Relying only on questions related to quantity and frequency of alcohol use may lead to underidentification of unhealthy alcohol use among older adults, given older adults' lower tolerance and the potential to experience adverse consequences at lower consumption levels. Therefore, in addition to questions about quantity and frequency, it can be helpful to ask about personal consequences of alcohol use and include a validated assessment of alcohol use. Validated measures for older adults are discussed later in this chapter (see Section 5.3 Choosing Appropriate Assessment Tools).

Screening strategies should take potential cultural differences into account. There are a number of screening measures that have been evaluated with racial and ethnic minority populations, including measures such as the Alcohol Use Disorders Identification Test – Consumption (AUDIT-C), which have been translated into multiple languages (see Manuel et al., 2015, for a review). When screening for unhealthy alcohol use with racial and ethnic minority clients, it is important to use culturally sensitive screening methods and make additional efforts to normalize routine screening as standard practice with all clients. Also consider the social determinants of health (e.g., stress because of discrimination) potentially associated with increased drinking in racial and ethnic minority populations, and the overall distrust that racial and ethnic minority clients may have for health care practitioners and systems owing to recent and historical experiences with racism and discrimination.

Screening, brief intervention, and referral to treatment (SBIRT) is a widely promoted approach to identification, assessment, and triage of unhealthy alcohol use (https://www.samhsa.gov/sbirt). SBIRT includes routine alcohol screening in medical or social service settings to detect unhealthy alcohol use, a brief discussion about alcohol and consequences of use, often integrating motivational interviewing (MI) techniques, as well as brief advice to cut back, and referral to specialty alcohol treatment if needed. This approach helps connect clients to alcohol treatment services, when indicated. SBIRT was developed as a universal screening approach and typically includes the AUDIT-C. For those who screen positive on the AUDIT-C pre-screen, additional assessment helps to determine severity level and understand specific alcohol-related problems. Clinical Vignette 1 demonstrates how screening can be incorporated into a clinical interview with an older client. The parenthetical text shows the key practitioner skills. Following the vignette, Table 8 summarizes the key screening recommendations covered in this section.

Clinical Vignette 1:
Incorporating screening into the clinical interview

Practitioner: If it's ok with you, I'd like to talk with you for a few minutes about your drinking patterns. This is a topic I raise with all of my clients. Would that be ok with you? (Normalize Screening and Asking Permission)

Client: Sure. I guess. I'm not worried about my drinking though. It's my sleep that I'm concerned about today.

Practitioner: Sleep is your number one priority today, and I definitely want to hear your concerns about your sleep. Sleep, mood, and health can also be impacted by drinking, so first, let's see if and how your drinking may be affecting your sleep. If you think about your drinking over the past month, how many days per week would you say that you typically drink alcohol? (Assess Drinking Patterns)

Client: I have a few glasses of wine each night. Usually I will have a glass or two with dinner and then maybe another one or two drinks after dinner. My spouse and I drink together and we don't get drunk or anything. We've drunk this way for 40 years. Actually, there were many periods where we were drinking a lot more!

Practitioner: This isn't a new pattern for you, and if anything, you've cut back over the years.

Client: Yes, that's right. I cut back because my spouse and I gained some weight. We were drinking a fair amount and feeling unhealthy. Our health is really important to us, and sleep has also become a big issue. Which is why I'm here today, I really want to get some help with my sleep. It's been off for a few months now. I wake up in the middle of the night and can't fall back to sleep.

Practitioner: Sleep is a huge concern for you. It's really impacting your life. Would it be ok if I shared some information about drinking and how it may impact your sleep? (Discuss Personal Consequences of Drinking)

Client: Ok.

Practitioner: I really appreciate all that you shared about your drinking. From what you told me, it seems like you might be drinking anywhere from 14 to 28 drinks a week. (Personal Feedback about Drinking)

Client: That seems like a lot! I guess when you add it up, yeah that seems about right.

Practitioner: It's surprising when you total it all up.

Client: Yeah, it's more than I thought. But it's not causing me any problems. I'm still doing my daily walks, even though I'm so tired from not sleeping.

Practitioner: Yeah, I can see that your health is really important to you. I'm not sure if this information will surprise you, but there is actually a well-known relationship between alcohol and sleep. Alcohol can cause you to feel drowsy, and some people say a few drinks help them fall asleep at night. But as the body continues to metabolize alcohol throughout the night, something called a rebound effect can occur, which causes you to wake up. So people who have been drinking actually wake up much more frequently throughout the night, and they don't feel as rested the next day. What do you make of this information? (Revisit Client-Generated Consequences)

Client: Well, that might be what is happening. I didn't realize alcohol could cause me to wake up more.

Practitioner: This is all new information for you. You've really enjoyed having a few glasses of wine each night, and now you're wondering if it may be contributing to your sleep problems.

Client: Yeah, if drinking is messing up my sleep, it's not worth it.

Practitioner: Sleep is definitely a priority for you. You're really considering making some changes to your drinking. Perhaps next we can talk about what that might look like for you. (Prepare to Make a Plan)

Table 8. Screening recommendations

Screening recommendation	Importance for older clients
Screen older adults at least yearly.	Unhealthy alcohol use often goes undetected, particularly among older adults.
Screen for unhealthy alcohol use in all settings.	Older adults receive services in multiple settings, including senior centers and assisted living facilities.
Screen all clients, including women and racial/ethnic minority clients.	Older women and those from racial/ethnic minority groups may be overlooked in screening.
Screen using the current guidelines.	Consider the NIAAA guidelines of no more than three drinks on any single day and no more than seven drinks per week for women, and no more than four drinks on any single day and no more than 14 drinks per week for men.

5.2 Assessment of Unhealthy Alcohol Use

Screening for unhealthy alcohol use helps to determine which clients are engaging in unhealthy alcohol use, in order to follow up with further assessment. Screening and assessment differ in that screening is typically brief and detects the presence of unhealthy alcohol use, whereas assessment is more comprehensive and evaluates the extent and specific characteristics of unhealthy alcohol use. Assessment can also inform a diagnosis and treatment plan, whereas screening typically does not provide enough information for a diagnosis.

Once unhealthy alcohol use has been identified, further assessment assists in understanding the history of the client's alcohol use, environmental factors, and impact on various levels of functioning. An assessment may be guided by DSM-5 criteria or may be less structured. Some factors to consider during assessment include comorbid health problems and the client's motivation to reduce or abstain from drinking. Important areas to cover related to alcohol use include alcohol and other substance use history, age of onset of alcohol-related problems, past and current amount and frequency of drinking, relationship of alcohol use to daily functioning, extent of substance use problems in the family, past attempts to limit or control alcohol intake, prior experiences with treatment, and history of any legal problems, especially those potentially related to alcohol use. Additional areas to explore include use of alcohol to manage pain, anxiety, or sleep problems. Other domains to cover in a comprehensive assessment include major medical conditions, current mental health symptoms and prior mental health diagnoses, relationship status, social support, and current living arrangements.

5.2.1 Assessing Medically Complex Older Adults

Older adults tend to have more chronic medical problems than other age groups and are more likely than younger age groups to use one or more prescription medications (Boersma et al., 2020). When assessing unhealthy alcohol use, practitioners should ask about current medical conditions and review a list of all prescription and over-the-counter medications. It can be easy to attribute symptoms of unhealthy alcohol use to a medical condition. For example, symptoms like confusion or falls could be attributed to diabetes or high blood pressure complications rather than a red flag for assessment of unhealthy alcohol use. Further, long-term alcohol use can cause or worsen medical conditions such as diabetes, high blood pressure, congestive heart failure, liver problems, osteoporosis, heart attack, and cerebrovascular changes. At the same time, multiple types of conditions, including unhealthy alcohol use, could be contributing to the client's current symptoms, which is why it is important to coordinate care with other members of the client's health care team.

> **Clinical Pearl**
>
> Poor management of chronic medical conditions may be an indicator of problematic alcohol use, such as by impacting the ability to follow medication instructions and follow up with providers about routine care. The threshold for unhealthy alcohol use may be lower among medically complex older adults.

More chronic medical conditions usually lead to the use of more prescription and over-the-counter medications. Using multiple medications (polypharmacy) increases the likelihood of drug–drug interactions. The problem with having multiple medications in the context of alcohol use is twofold. First, using a lot of different prescription drugs may make it difficult to follow the specific directions for each medication, thereby increasing the likelihood that medications are missed or taken more or less frequently than intended. This can lead to unintentional medication misuse. Second, having multiple medications makes it more likely that there will be an interaction between alcohol and medications (either individually or in combination). This may result in increased confusion, falls, motor problems, gastrointestinal distress, and other symptoms. Common medications that negatively interact with alcohol among older adults include aspirin, acetaminophen, cold and allergy medicine (antihistamines), cough syrup, sleeping medication, pain medication, anxiolytics, antihypertensives, and antidepressants (NIAAA, 2014). Consultation with the older adult's primary care physician may be warranted for older adults who screen positive for unhealthy alcohol use and have several prescription medications. Additionally, unhealthy alcohol use can also interfere with the ability to manage chronic medical conditions and take medications as indicated. Table 9 summarizes the key assessment recommendations from this section.

Table 9. Assessment recommendations

Assessment recommendations	Importance for older clients
Perform a comprehensive assessment across multiple domains of functioning.	Older adults may have a longer history of unhealthy alcohol use, and assessment needs to cover the full history of alcohol use. Other areas to assess include comorbid medical and mental health conditions, relationship status, social support, and current living situation.
Collect additional information when assessing medically complex older adults.	Older adults typically have one or more chronic health conditions that can be impacted by any alcohol use. Prescription and over-the-counter medications often interact negatively with any alcohol use. Collaboration with other members of the client's health care team can assist in determining the contribution of different conditions to the current symptoms.

5.3 Choosing Appropriate Assessment Tools

Use of valid, reliable, and accurate measures is essential when assessing for AUD. Unfortunately, validity and reliability are often based on specific research studies that may not include older adults. The validity, reliability, and accuracy of assessment may be compromised if a practitioner chooses measures that have not been validated with an older adult population. For example, older adults may experience alcohol-related symptoms differently when compared with adults in other age groups, or they may be experienced differently from the population on which the assessment was developed and normed.

Most alcohol assessment tools were not created specifically for older adults but were instead developed for a general adult population. As noted previously (see Section 4.1 DSM-5 Criteria for Alcohol Use Disorder), the symptoms that older adults experience related to alcohol use may not be severe enough to warrant a DSM-5 diagnosis (Kuerbis et al., 2013). This means that the same symptoms included in an assessment created for younger adults may not apply to the symptoms that older adults experience, or that a different (often lower) cutoff score may be necessary to correctly classify older adults with unhealthy alcohol use or AUDs. This section focuses on instruments validated in older populations or developed specifically with older clients in mind.

5.3.1 Alcohol Use Disorders Identification Test

The Alcohol Use Disorders Identification Test (AUDIT; Saunders et al., 1993) is a commonly used alcohol assessment, frequently used in health care settings. The full AUDIT (10 items) includes questions about alcohol intake (quantity, frequency, and binge drinking), alcohol-related consequences, and symptoms of dependence. Clients are also typically given a standard drinks chart to reference while answering questions (see Table 2). Items are scored on a scale from 0 to 4, and the total score ranges from 0 to 40. Scores between 1 and 7 reflect low-risk consumption, scores between 8 and 14 reflect harmful alcohol use, and scores greater than 15 suggest a high likelihood of a moderate to severe AUD. Based on this scoring system, a score of 8 or greater warrants additional assessment; however, prior research indicates that using a score of 8 produces low sensitivity (Aalto et al., 2011). The sensitivity of the AUDIT is increased when a cutoff score of 5 is used, and this lower cutoff score may be appropriate in working with older adults, given that lower levels of drinking may be associated with adverse consequences in this population.

Shorter versions of the AUDIT are useful in fast-paced clinical settings such as primary care. The AUDIT-C includes the three consumption questions of the AUDIT (quantity, frequency, and heavy episodic drinking) and is scored from 0 to 12 (see Appendix 3). The focus on quantity and frequency in the AUDIT-C may lead to lower scores for older adults, who do not need to drink as much to experience alcohol-related consequences. For these reasons, using the full AUDIT or the Short Michigan Alcoholism Screening Test – Geriatric Version (SMAST-G; discussed in the next section) may be more appropriate for older adults, since there is less of a focus on quantity and frequency. For the AUDIT-C, a score of 4 or more is considered positive for men; for women, a score of 3 or more is considered positive. In a study that evaluated the use of the AUDIT-C with residents of a nursing home, the accepted cutoff for men (4 or more) was supported, though the optimal cutoff for women was 2 or more (Dreher-Weber et al., 2017). In a comparison of the AUDIT, AUDIT-C, and *cutting down, annoyance, guilty feeling,* and *eye-*

openers (CAGE) set of questions, among adults aged 65 and older in a primary care clinic, the sensitivity of the AUDIT-C was 100 %, compared with 67 % for the AUDIT and 39 % for the CAGE questions (Gómez et al., 2006), indicating that the AUDIT-C may be the best choice for detecting unhealthy alcohol use among older adults.

There are also single-item versions of the AUDIT. Common items chosen for screening are Item 3 (AUDIT-3) regarding heavy episodic drinking or Item 4 (AUDIT-4) regarding whether the client can stop drinking once they start. Although the AUDIT performs well in a general adult population, the psychometric properties are not as strong in older adults (Källmén et al., 2014). Specifically, Items 1 and 4 (frequency and ability to stop drinking) were significantly less reliable and valid among older adults compared with the general adult population.

5.3.2 Michigan Alcoholism Screening Test – Geriatric Version – and Short MAST-G

The Michigan Alcoholism Screening Test – Geriatric Version (MAST-G) was developed specifically for older adults (Blow et al., 1991). It includes 24 yes or no items and was designed to account for differences in social and employment situations between younger and older adults. A score of 5 or more indicates likely unhealthy alcohol use. In a comparison of the MAST-G and the Fast Alcohol Screening Test (FAST), which is based on items from the AUDIT, the FAST failed to capture a significant number of older adults who had a history of unhealthy alcohol use (Knightly et al., 2016). In this study, the MAST-G was significantly more sensitive than the FAST. This result provides further evidence that using an alcohol assessment that was developed on younger adults may lead practitioners to miss older adults who have problems related to unhealthy alcohol use. The briefer Short MAST-G (SMAST-G) includes 10 yes or no items (see Appendix 4). A score of 2 or more is indicative of likely unhealthy alcohol use.

5.4 Conclusions: Screening and Assessment of Unhealthy Alcohol Use

All older adults should be screened yearly for unhealthy alcohol use, using a screening measure that is valid for an older adult population. Screening should occur across settings in the community to include older adults who may not routinely attend medical appointments. SBIRT is a common screening program and is effective for older adults (Schonfeld, 2020). If a screening measure is positive for unhealthy alcohol use, a more comprehensive assessment will assist in better understanding alcohol use patterns. Assessing medically complex older adults often involves a review of their medications and coordination of care in collaboration with their other medical providers.

6

Psychological Interventions

There are a number of evidence-based treatments for unhealthy alcohol use, but few have been designed and tested specifically with older adults (Kuerbis et al., 2014). Adults aged 65 and over are often excluded from clinical trials, thereby limiting the ability to evaluate effectiveness with them. Nonetheless, several interventions are well-suited for use with older adults. These treatments will be reviewed in this chapter, as well as general considerations for psychological interventions with older adults.

There is no one-size-fits-all approach to effectively addressing unhealthy alcohol use in older adults. The most recent SAMHSA Treatment Improvement Protocol (TIP) for substance use problems in older adults (SAMHSA, 2020) recommends that treatment for unhealthy alcohol use begin with a less intensive approach such as a brief intervention that integrates MI. For older adults with low-severity problems, treatment can be as short as one session focused on motivational interviewing (MI) and a few cognitive behavioral therapy (CBT) coping strategies, as discussed later in this chapter. Beginning with a less-intensive approach first is consistent with a stepped care model (Sobell & Sobell, 2000). Stepped care models deliver a more intensive treatment only to those individuals who do not experience noticeable improvement from less intensive interventions. Low-intensity interventions might include referral to 12-step or other mutual help groups (MHGs), personalized feedback about alcohol consumption, or brief interventions delivered in primary care. Individuals are typically only referred to specialty substance use services if indicated by the client's drinking levels or if the client does not benefit from less intensive forms of treatment. The components of stepped care are individualized to the client's strengths and resources. In addition, chosen interventions must be evidence-based, and should start with the least restrictive option likely to be effective based on assessment of the client's demographic and clinical characteristics.

In instances when a more intensive approach might be beneficial, practitioners can still start with a brief intervention focused on building motivation for engagement in longer, more intensive substance use interventions. More intensive treatment can involve providing more frequent or longer sessions, or may include switching to (or adding) other treatment options such as anticraving medications (see Chapter 7). For practitioners following a CBT approach, treatment can be expanded to include more CBT components. Section 6.6 on CBT in this chapter presents standard CBT techniques used in longer-term substance use treatments (e.g., identifying automatic thoughts and cognitive distortions) as well as techniques that are appropriate for a lower-severity client who could benefit from a brief three- to four-session treatment.

When selecting an appropriate treatment, it is important to consider severity of unhealthy alcohol use as well as medical and other conditions, and to explore client preferences (e.g., treatment delivery method, intensity, modality) when discussing options for care. Clients interested in treatment will often benefit from hearing about a variety of available treatment options (e.g., "There are a variety of choices available here. Let's review the different treatment options and see what seems like a good fit to you"). This process supports autonomy and helps the client make informed decisions about care.

Older adults may report different barriers to treatment for unhealthy alcohol use. For example, one study found that older adults reported barriers such as unreadiness to change, lack of knowledge about treatment options, and treatment availability, whereas adults in younger age groups (26–64 years) frequently mentioned cost as a barrier to treatment, followed by unreadiness to change, concerns about stigma and confidentiality, and the belief that they could manage their alcohol use on their own (Choi et al., 2014). In sum, low motivation to change and lack of information about treatment may hinder treatment engagement among older adults. This further highlights the relevance of motivational interventions combined with client education regarding the range of approaches that could be used to manage unhealthy alcohol use.

6.1 Care Coordination

Care coordination refers to sharing relevant information about clients to all members of the health care team to deliver safer and more effective care (Camicia et al., 2013). Care coordination is particularly important for older adults because they are often seeing multiple health care providers, including a primary care physician and specialists. Family members may also be involved in the older adult's health care. Behavioral interventions are increasingly provided in the context of integrated health care systems with shared medical records, but this is still far from standard in the US. Practitioners need to do whatever they can to minimize the chances of care becoming fragmented.

After obtaining appropriate releases, practitioners working in independent practice are encouraged to contact other current health care providers to talk with them about their assessment of the client's alcohol use and treatment goals. This conversation can also assist in differential diagnosis – for example, by clarifying how symptoms of the client's medical conditions overlap with symptoms of unhealthy alcohol use. This information is particularly useful for medically complex older adults who may have symptoms resulting from multiple conditions, including unhealthy alcohol use. Through this process practitioners can also gain insights into whether and how the client describes their alcohol use to other providers or family members.

6.2   Treatment Modifications for Older Adults

There are several ways in which treatment may need to be modified for older adults. For example, practitioners may require additional information on how to assess and accommodate visual and cognitive impairments in older adults, and how generational experiences associated with being in a particular birth cohort (e.g., Baby Boomers) might play a role in treatment. These issues are explored below.

Practitioners should be aware of older adults' potential generational stigma concerning treatment for unhealthy alcohol use as well as mental health treatment more broadly (Slade et al., 2016). In prior generations of older adults, it was uncommon to seek treatment for unhealthy alcohol use and was also looked down upon as a sign of weakness or failure. Thus, treatment may need to be adapted to reduce the perceived stigma of seeking help for unhealthy alcohol use. As an example of language that reduces stigma, older adults tend to prefer more neutral language in therapeutic encounters (e.g., class and teacher) rather than language that indicates treatment for a disorder (Center for Substance Abuse Treatment, 2005). Additionally, further time may need to be spent in the rapport-building phase with older adults. This additional time may assist the practitioner in better understanding generational perspectives and values that an older client brings to treatment for unhealthy alcohol use.

The SAMHSA TIP for older adults (SAMHSA, 2020) also offers guidance on age-sensitive treatment for unhealthy alcohol use among older adults. Their recommendations include a focus on supportive and nonconfrontational interventions, flexibility in how services are delivered (such as by phone or in the home vs. at an office), and sensitivity to gender differences, especially since older women are more likely to be prescribed psychoactive medications that may interact with alcohol. Other recommendations include providing materials in the client's preferred language, sensitivity to the client's potential mobility limitations and other aspects of physical functioning, providing an intervention that is holistic and thorough, and choosing interventions that focus on developing and improving coping and social skills.

With regard to physical functioning, practitioners should consider factors like office location in relation to the building entrance. For example, how much walking will an older client have to do to get to the office from the parking lot, and how many steps there are to enter the building. Practitioners should conduct sessions in a well-lit office and provide clients with high-contrast printed materials (black font on white paper) in a slightly larger font (14 pt) to accommodate age-related vision changes. When completing assessments, providing a response card with the relevant scale anchors can help cue older adults to response options throughout the assessment phase. There are other strategies that can be used to promote retention of information across sessions, which may be particularly important for older adults with cognitive impairment. Caution is warranted to not engage in ageism around these modifications by slowing down or repeating information when it is not needed. The strategies suggested by SAMHSA (2020) for increasing retention of information include:

- Summarizing and repeating information throughout the session and at the end of the session. This summary might include specific insights that the client had, as well as new skills learned during sessions.
- Suggest that the older client take notes during sessions. Alternatively, the practitioner can prepare a set of notes about the session that the client can take home. As appropriate, involving family members can be helpful so that they can understand the skills that the client is learning in sessions.
- Offer handouts, reminder calls, and forms. This increases the likelihood that the client will complete tasks between sessions and arrive at sessions on time. Research with older adults has shown that homework compliance significantly improves posttreatment outcomes (Coon & Thompson, 2003).
- Consider increasing the number of sessions offered so that the pacing of each session is not rushed. This reduces the demands within each session such that information is more spread out across sessions.

Other situations that practitioners may experience when working with older adult clients include mobility and transportation problems. Flexibility and problem solving are required for mobility and transportation problems. This may include use of telehealth sessions (i.e., phone or video) or arranging transportation with a caregiver if transportation and mobility difficulties are barriers to in-person treatment sessions. Because of the COVID-19 pandemic, older clients may have more comfort with telehealth, and this format may improve access to services, particularly for individuals in rural areas. Telehealth may be preferred for some older adults owing to the ease of access and ability to control audio quality through speakers or a headset.

6.3 Harm Reduction Versus Abstinence-Based Treatments

Harm reduction involves taking steps to reduce the risk associated with alcohol use but not completely eliminating drinking, whereas *abstinence-based approaches* aim to eliminate alcohol use altogether. For example, harm reduction for older adults may include reduction to low-risk drinking within the limits for recommended alcohol consumption (no more than three drinks per day and no more than seven drinks per week for women; no more than four drinks per day and 14 drinks per week for men). Harm reduction has increased in popularity in recent decades, partially because the natural course of alcohol use across the adult lifespan includes reduction of use over time rather than full abstinence (Peele, 2016), and because clients often prefer harm reduction over abstinence.

There is a significant amount of research on harm reduction among younger and middle-aged adults, but harm reduction outcomes among older adults are not well-represented in the literature. Han (2019) suggests that a harm reduction approach is consistent with the principles of chronic disease management and geriatric medical care, as compared with an abstinence-based approach. For example, the principles for medical care for older adults who are medically complex include (1) eliciting and incorporating client preferences and goals into medical decision making, (2) less of a focus on "cures or fixes" and more of a focus on meaningful outcomes for older clients, and (3) making practical and incremental changes. Therefore, geriatricians (and other providers working with older adults who follow this approach) become accustomed to working within a harm reduction model whereby risks are mitigated, but not completely eliminated, through shared decision making. Some progress toward wellness is considered better than no progress, and the goal is not necessarily to "fix" the problem. Therefore, there is already high overlap with the principles of harm reduction versus abstinence in the field of geriatric medicine.

In sum, it is worth considering whether a harm reduction approach focused on low-risk drinking is appropriate for a client. Specific harm reduction strategies might include alternating between alcoholic and nonalcoholic drinks during a drinking session, making sure not to drink on an empty stomach, switching to drinks with lower alcohol content, and taking extra precautions to avoid adverse medication interactions. Assessing client preferences for harm reduction versus abstinence and consideration of whether their alcohol use history and problem severity fits better with one approach or the other can be part of the initial clinical interview process to develop a collaborative treatment plan.

6.4 Brief Interventions

Brief interventions such as MI are useful in exploring a client's ambivalence and potential reasons for change. Brief interventions are associated with reductions in drinking (Ettner et al., 2014; Moore et al., 2011; Schonfeld et al., 2010) and are often effective as a stand-alone intervention for those with low-severity unhealthy alcohol use. Brief interventions may be all that is needed for those with low to moderate alcohol consumption, whereas those with more severe problems may require more extensive treatment. In a traditional (i.e., longer-term) psychotherapy context, brief interventions may be relevant if low-severity unhealthy alcohol use is detected, but alcohol use is not the primary treatment target. There are multiple ways to define the content and length of treatments that are labeled as brief interventions. For example, with clients in the low-severity range on measures of alcohol use, the practitioner can engage the client in a brief exploration of current alcohol use and potential risks, and advise the client to reduce drinking. This approach is often referred to as "brief advice" and has been widely used in primary care, mental health, and other settings. Consistent with the SBIRT approach, this is typically a one-time discussion about alcohol use and includes the steps outlined in Box 2.

Box 2. Brief advice steps in the SBIRT approach

1. Explain to the client that they are drinking over recommended limits.
2. Advise the client to cut back according to the low-risk drinking guidelines (no more than three drinks on any 1 day and no more than seven drinks per week for women; no more than four drinks per day and 14 per week for men).
3. Connect this advice to potential health risks or to consequences that the client is already experiencing from unhealthy alcohol use.

Note. SBIRT = screening, brief intervention, and referral to treatment.

It is generally a good idea to meet with the client during subsequent sessions to see if changes were made and to reinforce the importance of cutting back on drinking. If a client has not made any changes in response to the brief advice intervention, or if the client is in the moderate- to high-risk category for unhealthy alcohol use upon screening, they may benefit from a brief alcohol-focused treatment. There are several options for brief treatments, which are typically defined as four or fewer group or individual sessions. The most recent SAMHSA TIP for substance use problems in older adults (SAMHSA, 2020) outlines a brief semistructured interview format that can be used if practitioners determine that an older client is engaging in unhealthy alcohol use and needs additional intervention (Box 3).

Box 3. SAMHSA Treatment Improvement Protocol (TIP) brief intervention

1. Start the conversation by asking about future goals in multiple areas, including health, activities, hobbies, and relationships. This information can be helpful for Step 5, when the practitioner explores the client's reasons for cutting back on alcohol use.
2. Give the client feedback on their level of alcohol use and discuss how it compares with the low-risk drinking guidelines.
3. Discuss the pros and cons of drinking, for the client. This may include a discussion of whether alcohol is helpful in coping with loss, loneliness, or other negative emotional states.
4. Provide information about the impact of unhealthy alcohol use on physical health, mental health, and social functioning. The practitioner should specify that these negative effects can occur even when an older adult drinks within recommended limits, because of increased sensitivity and lower tolerance for alcohol.
5. Discuss some reasons the client might have for cutting down on drinking. Common motivators for cutting back on use among older adults can include maintaining independence, physical health, and cognitive abilities.
6. Offer information about how the older client could cut down, such as by engaging in other social activities or hobbies.
7. Create a plan that includes drinking limits agreed upon with the client. It may be helpful to ask the client to sign this agreement.
8. Discuss high-risk drinking situations. For older adults, these situations may include loneliness, boredom, and difficult interactions with family.
9. Conclude the brief intervention by summarizing the session.

Note. SAMHSA = US Substance Abuse and Mental Health Services Administration.

Several brief treatment models for older adults have been developed and tested in primary care settings. Examples include Project Guiding Older Adult Lifestyles (Project GOAL; Fleming et al., 1999), Healthy Living as You Age (Moore et al., 2011), and Project Senior Health and Alcohol Risk Education (Project SHARE; Ettner et al., 2014). These interventions commonly consist of an assessment followed by a few short sessions focused on MI, recognizing drinking triggers and antecedents, and strategies for managing urges (discussed further in Section 6.6 Cognitive Behavioral Therapy). As an example, Project GOAL (Fleming et al., 1999) included a short assessment interview along with a workbook containing information on health

behaviors, and review of problem drinking prevalence, drinking antecedents, cues, and adverse effects. Additionally, participants were asked to track
their alcohol use on drinking diary cards. In two follow-up appointments
with their physician (10–15 minutes each), intervention condition participants received personalized feedback about their alcohol use, and an alcohol consumption agreement was created and given to the client in the form
of a prescription. Participants received a phone call after each office visit.
The components of these primary care–based brief treatments, including
goal setting, daily tracking of alcohol use, and identification of triggers, antecedents, and consequences of unhealthy alcohol use, can be helpful for
practitioners working in a range of settings including those based in social
services or independent counseling practices.

Brief interventions generally have several aspects in common. First, they
consist of approximately three to four sessions. Second, they are intended
for clients with low-severity problems who are not experiencing major consequences of alcohol use. Third, they generally focus on a combination of
MI and CBT techniques, including exploration of reasons for reducing alcohol use. Clients may be asked to self-monitor alcohol use on a daily basis
to understand patterns of use. Using this information, clients are asked to
identify triggers and antecedents for alcohol use, as well as consequences
of use. Following this, specific skills may be introduced that focus on determining alternative activities for high-risk alcohol use situations, or other
problem-solving skills such as managing anxiety or depressed mood. Finally, prevention skills are introduced to help the client develop a plan to
manage future cravings and slips.

6.5   Motivational Interviewing

Motivational interviewing (MI) is a collaborative, client-centered approach
(Miller & Rollnick, 2013) that is widely used to address a variety of health
behaviors, both harmful, including alcohol and other substance use, and
healthy, such as exercise, healthy eating, and medical treatment adherence
(Frost et al., 2018; Rubak et al., 2005). MI is effective as a stand-alone brief
intervention for unhealthy alcohol use (e.g., one or two sessions) in both
mental health and medical settings. Additionally, MI may be used as a pre-
cursor to enhance motivation for other longer, more intensive treatment
modalities (e.g., longer-term CBT).

In MI, discussions about behavior change occur within a framework of
nonjudgmental acceptance, empathic listening, and partnership between
the practitioner and client. MI practitioners seek to understand the client's
perspective, with the goal of eliciting the client's potential reasons for mak-

ing a behavior change. MI theory views behavior change as an individualized process in which eliciting a client's own values and perspectives enhances the likelihood of subsequent behavior change – versus the practitioner telling clients what to do (Miller & Rollnick, 2013). In this vein, MI practitioners avoid directing or instructing a client on the change process, in favor of a collaborative guiding process. A key premise in MI is that pushing or coercing clients, particularly ambivalent clients, into a behavior change will likely lead to increased client resistance to change, arguing for things to stay as they are (e.g., continued unhealthy alcohol use). The more a client defends the status quo, the less likely they are to change their behavior.

MI is best-suited for clients who are ambivalent about engaging in a particular behavior change (e.g., reducing their alcohol consumption). MI practitioners approach behavior change discussions with the understanding that ambivalence is a normal and expected part of the behavioral change process. Ambivalent clients will naturally voice both their reasons to change (e.g., "I am tired of feeling hungover every morning.") and their reasons not to change ("I've had cocktails at the end of the day for 40 years. It's who I am"). This focus on client language is central to MI. Client language is categorized into *change talk* and *sustain talk* (see Table 10 for examples). Client change talk includes client statements of the reasons, desire, ability, need, and commitment to change whereas sustain talk includes language consistent with maintaining the status quo (e.g., continued drinking).

Prior studies of MI have demonstrated a relationship between practitioner within-session skills (e.g., open questions, affirmations, reflections), client language (change and sustain talk), and treatment outcomes (Catley et al., 2006; Magill et al., 2018). These studies have found that when practitioners ask open-

Table 10. Examples of client change talk and sustain talk

Client language	Change talk	Sustain talk
Desire	I want to cut back on my drinking.	I don't want to be a teetotaler.
Ability	I could cut drinking during the week.	I don't think I can quit.
Reasons	The calories are really adding up for me.	I like to have a few glasses of wine when I see my friends.
Need	I need to get my drinking under control.	I don't see a need to make any changes right now.
Commitment	I am going to stop buying alcohol. It will help if I don't have it at home.	I'm not interested in changing right now. Maybe at some point, but not now.

ended questions about a behavior change (e.g., "Why did your partner say he is worried about your drinking?"), affirm the patient ("You've thought a lot about the different ways you could cut back on drinking"), and reflect client change talk ("He's concerned that you might fall again when you're drinking"), clients are likely to respond with additional change talk statements. Furthermore, studies have demonstrated a relationship between within-session client language and subsequent treatment outcomes (Magill & Hallgren, 2019). The role of client sustain talk has emerged as particularly important, with higher levels of within-session sustain talk predicting worse treatment outcomes across a number of studies. Thus, in MI, practitioners seek to strategically elicit and reflect client change talk in a collaborative, empathic, and autonomy-supportive manner. Although client sustain talk is expected in discussions about behavior change with ambivalent clients, MI practitioners will often avoid a direct focus on eliciting and reinforcing sustain talk.

Key MI techniques include the use of open-ended questions, affirmations, autonomy-supportive statements, reflections, and summaries (see Table 11, for examples and definitions). Reflective listening, or conveying an understanding of a client's perspective, is a core skill in MI. Skilled MI practitioners will offer twice as many reflections as questions in any given MI interaction. Reflections are categorized into *simple reflections* (repeating or rephrasing what a client has said) and *complex reflections* that go beyond what a client has directly said and often reflect the underlying emotion in a client statement (see examples in Table 12). Summary statements are a compilation of client statements presented together and are often used to end an MI interaction or transition to a different topic. Clinical Vignette 2 demonstrates key MI techniques in the parenthetical text, using the same older client introduced in prior chapters.

Clinical Vignette 2: The key techniques of MI

Practitioner: Earlier, we spoke about the ways drinking might be affecting your sleep. You were pretty surprised to hear that alcohol can cause difficulties with sleep. You even mentioned that drinking wasn't worth it if it's interfering with your sleep. (Summary)

Client: Don't get me wrong, I like to drink and really don't think it's that big of a deal. It's not like I've gotten arrested while drinking or anything. (Sustain Talk) But when you said that it might be contributing to my sleep problems, I realized a few glasses of wine at night aren't worth a restless night of sleep. (Change Talk)

Practitioner: You're not happy about potentially making a change in your drinking. And at the same time, you're concerned about these sleep problems. (Complex Reflection)

Client: Yes, I've been thinking about whether I should take a break. I figure it's worth taking a week or two off from drinking to see how it affects my sleep. (Change Talk)

Practitioner: You want to test this out and see if you sleep better when you're not drinking. (Complex Reflection) How might you go about taking a week off from drinking? What would that look like for you? (Open-ended Question)

Client: I don't know. I'm not addicted to alcohol or anything but it's definitely a big part of my evening routine. (Sustain Talk)

Practitioner: It's hard to imagine what taking a week off from drinking would even look like. (Complex Reflection)

Client: Yeah, it is a big shift.

Practitioner: You feel two ways about it. On the one hand, this is a big change, and you're not sure what it will even look like. At the same time, you are really concerned about your sleep. You want to be sleeping better. (Complex Reflection)

Client: Yeah, not sleeping is really affecting me. (Change Talk) So what should I do? Are you going to tell me to go to some long-term treatment program?

Practitioner: No, not at all. I can talk through the options with you, but this decision is completely up to you. (Emphasizing Autonomy)

Client: Well, I want to do something that makes sense to me. I don't want to feel forced into anything.

Practitioner: I hear that. This has to be your decision and it needs to make sense to you. (Emphasizing Autonomy)

Client: Yes, and once I decide to do something, I get it done.

Practitioner: You're the type of person who works hard to make change happen. (Affirmation) Well, let's talk through a couple of options and see what makes sense to you. One option is to keep meeting with me, one on one, for probably about 10 sessions. We can talk about coping strategies, things you can do when you feel pulled to drink. There are also groups, such as group therapy or self-help groups, like AA. What do you think about those options? (Open-ended Question)

Client: Individual therapy, with you, might be a good option. (Change Talk)

Practitioner: That seems like a good option to help you drink less and sleep better. (Simple Reflection)

Client: Yeah, I'm willing to give it a shot.

Practitioner: Great, well let's plan to meet next week at the same time, and we can start talking about next steps.

Hanson and Gutheil (2004) describe why MI may be particularly well-suited to older adults. Unhealthy alcohol use among older adults is often detected in non-addiction treatment settings and is often not the primary problem for which an older adult has sought care. If an older adult client does not appear motivated to change their drinking, MI tools can be used to explore potential reasons to cut back. In addition, MI's focus on empathy and self-efficacy may be appealing to older adults who frequently get messages from society and the health care system that they are not competent or that they need to do what the provider tells them without having much discussion. MI emphasizes individual autonomy. A collaborative style, focus on client strengths, and the underlying assumption that clients can make decisions for themselves about next steps are values consistent with what older adults need and appreciate in a health care provider.

MI also offers specific techniques especially appropriate to older adults. The use of open-ended questions, affirmations, autonomy-supportive statements, reflections, and summaries are consistent with the literature on the effectiveness of life-review and reminiscence therapies for older adults, treatments which allow clients to talk about their identity and age-related changes using their own words and experiences (Rubin et al., 2019). Because of ageism and other factors, older adults do not often have the experience of having someone's undivided attention. MI allows clients to have input in setting the pace of sessions. Finally, practitioners who practice MI tend to use reflections that integrate the client's own words when describing problems. Given that many older adults are not seeking care specifically for unhealthy alcohol use, use of labels ("alcoholic") may serve to reduce interest in treatment and further alienate older adults from receiving substance use and mental health services.

Through the process of exploring reasons for change and eliciting change talk, the practitioner can direct the conversation toward exploration of different steps that the client may consider. At this stage, an MI change plan worksheet can be used to guide treatment planning or behavior change discussions (see Table 13). This worksheet should only be incorporated into discussions when a client indicates willingness to move toward behavior change. Introducing this worksheet prematurely is likely to result in increased client sustain talk and feelings of coercion to engage in a behavior change. If clients have a negative reaction, revisit current motivation and ambivalence before proceeding further.

Table 11. Key motivational interviewing (MI) techniques

	Open-ended question	Affirmations	Autonomy-supportive statements	Reflections	Summaries
Definition	A question that elicits client response beyond a one- to two-word answer.	Statements that recognize client skills, behaviors, strengths.	Statements that highlight the client's choice and control.	Conveys understanding of what the client has said. Reflection is offered as a statement, without any inflection at the end of the statement.	Reflections of a few of the client's ideas or statements.
Examples	What are your thoughts about your drinking?	You are determined to make this happen.	You are worried that you might fall again.	You have worked really hard to make these changes.	You are worried about your drinking and can see it has increased lately. You aren't sure about next steps but know you need to make a change of some sort.
	How might things be different if you cut back on your drinking?		You've thought about cutting back.	You are determined to make this change.	You can see the benefits of cutting back. You'll feel better, spend less money, and your kids won't worry about you.

6 Psychological Interventions 57

Table 12. Simple and complex reflections

Client statement	Simple reflection	Complex reflection
Sure, I should probably cut back on my drinking a bit, but I'm not going to quit entirely.	You're not going to quit drinking entirely. You know you should probably cut back on your drinking.	You're not ready to give drinking up altogether and at the same time, it's clear that you need to make some changes.
What does treatment look like here? Is it a bunch of teenagers who got in trouble for smoking weed?	You're wondering what treatment looks like here.	You are curious about treatment options and want to find one that meets your needs.
My doctor tells me to quit drinking now, after 50 years of drinking this way.	You've been drinking this way for a long time.	Drinking has been a big part of your life over the years and you're surprised that your doctor is worried about it.

Table 13. Example change plan worksheet

Change plan worksheet

The changes I want to make are:

The most important reasons why I want to make these changes are:

The steps I plan to take in changing are:

The ways other people can help me are:	Person:
	Possible ways to help:

I will know that my plan is not working if:

I will know that my plan is working if:

6.6 Cognitive Behavioral Therapy

A *cognitive behavioral therapy* (CBT) model of psychotherapy for unhealthy alcohol use largely focuses on helping clients understand antecedents and consequences that are maintaining their current level of drinking (McCrady & Epstein, 2021). An overarching assumption is that drinking occurs in direct response to antecedents (factors that reliably precede alcohol use) and is maintained by its consequences. Antecedents and consequences can occur in multiple domains (see Table 3). Consequences can serve to reinforce alcohol use because of either the addition of positive experiences or the removal of negative experiences. The CBT model assumes that one way in which unhealthy alcohol use develops is through the repeated use of alcohol in certain situations, places, times of day, or emotional states. Over time, by using alcohol repeatedly in these situations, the client develops cravings to use alcohol in these trigger situations. Once an antecedent occurs, cognitions and affective status may determine the extent to which the antecedent leads to drinking behavior. For example, individuals may develop unhelpful beliefs about their ability to reduce drinking ("cutting down is not possible for me" or "I really would miss drinking if I stopped") which may lead to heavier drinking behavior compared with situations in which those beliefs are not activated.

CBT is readily adaptable to clients' individual contexts and beliefs around alcohol use. Practitioners may prefer the CBT approach for unhealthy alcohol use because it can be customized to focus on issues that are relevant to older adults (loneliness, health problems, etc.). There is also flexibility to customize treatment based on the appropriateness of cognitive versus behavioral techniques. There are many specific techniques that can be used within CBT treatment, and practitioners can tailor CBT by selecting primarily behavioral components, primarily cognitive components, or both.

For clients with low-severity problems where a single session may be appropriate, such as in health care settings, practitioners can use simple behavioral techniques such as asking the client to self-monitor alcohol intake. It may also be appropriate to give normative feedback to low-severity clients, such as the data by Chan and colleagues (2007) which found that the majority of older adults had zero or one drink per week and a minority of older adults were drinking above the NIAAA guidelines of no more than three drinks per day and seven drinks per week for women and no more than four drinks per day and 14 per week for men. If an older adult is drinking more than this, discussing the normative data may help the older client realize that they are drinking above the amount typically consumed by other older adults.

For clients who could use a few additional treatment sessions in the context of a brief intervention (three to four sessions), practitioners can introduce a *functional analysis*. This involves working with the client to identify the chain of events that leads to alcohol use through the identification of antecedents and consequences of alcohol use. A functional analysis helps clients understand how alcohol use functions in the context of the client's life and can help the client replace or reduce alcohol use with other behaviors. A functional analysis can also help the client identify high-risk situations that are likely to lead to alcohol use.

There are many ways that a functional analysis can be introduced. One option is that practitioners can introduce the ABC model, which stands for *antecedent, behavior,* and *consequences*. To demonstrate the ABC model, clients can be asked to identify a recent situation where they engaged in unhealthy alcohol use. The practitioner can help the client identify what was happening before alcohol use started and what occurred after. By engaging in this exercise, clients will begin to identify patterns in their alcohol use. For example, a client may realize that they typically drink when they are experiencing social anxiety. In this case, the antecedent may be going to a gathering on their own where they do not know anyone, in combination with nervousness. The behavior is excessive drinking, and the consequence is a hangover the next day. Another possible example of the ABC model is shown in Table 14 for drinking to cope with loneliness.

A functional analysis can help clients identify high-risk trigger or antecedent situations for alcohol use. For older adults, possible antecedents include a lack of enjoyable activities, loneliness, or social pressure associated with living in retirement communities in which drinking offers a means of interacting with others (Kuerbis et al., 2014). For some older adults, retirement leads to fewer opportunities for social interaction and meaningful activity. In this context, retirement can be a positive or negative antecedent. Retirement may bring increased leisure time but also loss of supportive social relationships from work and other social contexts. These factors can increase the risk of drinking more than intended.

Once alcohol use patterns are identified through a functional analysis, practitioners can work with clients to identify behaviors that can replace al-

Table 14. ABC model for alcohol use

Antecedent	Behavior	Consequences
Dave is sorting through boxes and finds photos from friends and family that he is no longer in touch with.	Dave feels lonely and drinks more than he usually does.	While drinking, Dave feels a little less sad about losing touch with old friends. The next morning he wakes up feeling groggy and finds it hard to start the day.

cohol use in high-risk situations. This can also be done in the context of a brief intervention. One option is to work with the client to increase situations in which they are engaging in alternative, rewarding behaviors that do not involve alcohol use. Behavioral activation is a specific behavioral strategy that targets increasing alternative behaviors and is used successfully with older adults with depression (Orgeta et al., 2017). This is sometimes referred to as *pleasant events scheduling*, and the goal is to increase the client's engagement in enjoyable, nondrinking activities such as spending time with family or friends, doing exercise, watching movies, doing hobbies, or any other activity that clients find enjoyable.

Clinical Pearl

Older adults' hobbies and interests may change in response to health concerns or other limitations, retirement, or other life changes. A pleasant events schedule for older adults, the California Older Person's Pleasant Event Schedule, presents activities that older adults tend to enjoy (Rider et al., 2016). Clients rate how often they engaged in the activity in the past month and how enjoyable the activity was or would be. Practitioners can then work with clients to increase participation in activities that are enjoyable but that they have not done lately.

The CBT strategies reviewed so far are an appropriate intervention for older clients with low-severity or mild problems who could benefit from a brief intervention (three to four sessions). These strategies include monitoring alcohol use, providing normative data on alcohol consumption among nationally representative samples of older adults, identifying triggers or antecedents for alcohol use, and working to replace alcohol use with other enjoyable activities, either through pleasant events scheduling or increasing social support. These strategies can be used together or separately depending on the client's situation. Emphasizing the behavioral components of CBT may be particularly useful for older adults with cognitive impairment, including adverse effects on memory that can result from long-term alcohol use. The behavioral strategies discussed in this section are summarized in Table 15.

For clients who need additional sessions owing to more severe unhealthy alcohol use, practitioners may wish to introduce the cognitive components of the CBT model, as well as more skills for managing triggers, recognizing cravings and urges, and practicing drink refusal skills (DeMarce et al., 2014). Coping skills can focus on both behavioral and cognitive strategies to manage high-risk situations and avoid drinking. Behavioral skills might include practicing how to engage in other coping strategies besides alcohol use, such

6 Psychological Interventions 61

Table 15. Behavioral components of treatment for older adults

Treatment goal	Description	Specific questions to assess
Self-monitoring alcohol use	The client tracks all alcohol use in a typical week.	Provide a blank form for the client to use throughout the week. Identify patterns of alcohol use.
Identifying drinking triggers and antecedents (functional analysis)	The practitioner can ask about specific situations, individuals, time of day, or emotions that usually precede alcohol use.	1. "Describe situations in the past when you were most likely to drink too much." 2. Ask questions about alcohol use that cover social, environmental, emotional, cognitive, and physical triggers. For example: "Who did you drink with last?" (social) "Where do you typically drink?" (environmental) "What mood are you typically in prior to drinking?" (emotional) "What thoughts do you typically have before drinking?" (cognitive) "Were you experiencing pain or other physical symptoms before drinking?" (physical)
Behavioral activation	This is sometimes referred to as *pleasant events scheduling*. Behavioral activation provides alternative, rewarding activities (replacement behaviors) during the times when alcohol use is most common. It can also be used to identify pleasant events that can replace alcohol use as a coping mechanism for negative emotions (e.g., calling a friend instead of drinking, in response to loneliness or boredom).	1. "What are some hobbies or other activities that you enjoy doing now or enjoyed doing at some point in your life?" 2. "When was the last time you did those hobbies?" From this point, the practitioner could use the California Older Person's Pleasant Events Schedule to determine additional pleasant events (see https://sgec.stanford.edu/content/dam/sm/sgec/documents/resources/Depression/OPPES%20-%20Pleasant%20Events.pdf).

62   Unhealthy Alcohol Use in Older Adults

Table 15.   continued

Treatment goal	Description	Specific questions to assess
Increasing social support	The practitioner may help the client to think about friends and family members in their current social network and explore ways to improve skills for developing or strengthening connections with others, especially individuals who are supportive of the client's efforts to cut down or eliminate drinking. This may include problem solving around how to reach out to friends and family and inviting them to specific events or activities, or trying new activities in order to make new social contacts.	1. "Tell me about your close friends and family." 2. "How often do you see close friends and family?"

Table 16.   Example of a three-column thought record

Situation	Thought	Feeling
Describe the individual, place, or thing that triggered the urge or craving.	Write down any automatic thoughts (or self-talk) you had about drinking.	What feeling(s) did you experience?
I met up with some old friends from work that I used to drink with.	This is fun. I'm glad I ran into them. Why did I stop getting drinks with them?	Excited. A little nervous about how much everyone will drink tonight.

as meeting up with a friend or engaging in a preferred pleasant event. Behavioral skills could also include practicing how to refuse an alcoholic drink in a social situation. Cognitive skills might include strategies for managing negative mood states, such as challenging cognitive distortions and replacing them with more neutral thoughts.

With regard to challenging cognitions, practitioners can first ask clients to keep a *thought record* to identify thoughts that occur in drinking situations. This is sometimes referred to as a *three-column thought record* (see Table 16, for example). The three columns are typically: (1) *situation* (individual, place, or thing that triggered the urge to drink), (2) *thought* (the client writes down any automatic thoughts or self-talk they had about drinking, and (3) *feeling* (emotions experienced during the situation). This thought record can assist with identifying common cognitive distortions that the client uses by examining any themes in the automatic thoughts or self-talk. From there, the practitioner can begin to gently challenge the identified cognitive distortions and help the client learn to do this for themselves.

Cognitive distortions are unhelpful thinking patterns that make it difficult to see a situation clearly and can lead to depressed or anxious mood or overreliance on alcohol. Examples include overgeneralizations, personalization or blame, black-and-white thinking, or catastrophizing. *Overgeneralization* occurs when a client comes to a negative conclusion that goes beyond the current situation. *Personalization* or *blame* occurs when a client thinks that another person's behavior is because of them and not related to other possible circumstances. For example, a driver honking at a client may lead the client to think that the driver is upset at them specifically, when in fact, the driver may be rushing to an emergency or honking for other factors. *Black-and-white thinking,* also called all-or-nothing thinking, occurs when a situation is viewed in two categories (good or bad) instead of on a continuum. *Catastrophizing* occurs when a client anticipates that future outcomes will be bad while discounting the likelihood of other, positive or more likely outcomes. These are just a few of the unhelpful thought patterns that individuals commonly have, which can function as cognitive triggers for alcohol use.

The goal of treatment when focusing on cognitive distortions is to understand the client's unhelpful thinking patterns and work to transition those thinking patterns into more balanced assessments of situations. For example, the beliefs that "I can't relax without alcohol" or that "My friends won't want to spend time with me unless I'm drinking alcohol" can be explored and gently challenged, and alternative ways of thinking proposed. This process is known as *cognitive restructuring*.

Here are some approaches that practitioners can use with clients to challenge cognitive distortions and automatic thoughts (DeMarce et al., 2014):
1. Ask the client to examine how realistic the automatic thought is. Is this thought based on facts or feelings?
2. Help the client find evidence for and against the automatic thought. What is the evidence that this thought is true? Is this thought out of habit or is it supported by facts?
3. Increase the client's flexibility in thinking about the situation. Is this situation black or white, or does it seem more complicated? Would others interpret this situation differently? Here, the practitioner could ask the client to consider what a friend would do in a similar situation.

Cognitive restructuring enables the client to challenge their own automatic thoughts, a practice that takes practice both in and outside of sessions. Use of a five-column thought record can be helpful here, which adds two additional columns to the three-column record: (4) *alternative realistic thought* (client uses the three questions listed previously to come up with a more balanced and realistic thought), and (5) *outcome* (client decides what feeling would result from using the alternative and more realistic thought; see Table 17, for example).

Table 17. Example of a five-column thought record

Situation	Thought	Feeling	Alternative, realistic thought	Outcome
Describe the individual, place, or thing that triggered the urge or craving.	Write down any automatic thoughts (or self-talk) you had about drinking.	What feeling(s) did you experience?	Come up with a more balanced, realistic thought.	What feeling or behavior might result from the alternative, realistic thought?
I met up with some old friends from work that I used to drink with.	This is fun. I'm glad I ran into them. Why did I stop getting drinks with them?	Excited. A little nervous about how much everyone will drink tonight.	Those times weren't that fun, and I usually drank too much. I'd wake up feeling pretty bad.	I'll enjoy their company and leave before the drinking starts.

Another common skill taught in CBT is managing cravings and urges to drink. Practitioners can start this component of treatment by highlighting that cravings are common, predictable, time-limited, and controllable (DeMarce et al., 2014). If the client has already identified triggers for alcohol use, it can be helpful to use their specific triggers to connect to the experience of cravings. For example, cravings may occur when experiencing pain (physical trigger) or loneliness (emotional trigger). Older clients can monitor cravings by writing down urges to use alcohol and describing what was happening directly before the urge started. Practitioners can use this information to talk through potential ways to manage cravings, such as engaging in an alternative activity or reaching out to a supportive friend or family member to talk.

Practitioners can also review drink refusal skills with clients. Clients experience direct social pressure in social gatherings when someone offers them a drink. Indirect social pressure occurs when a drink is not specifically offered, but the client thinks that they should have a drink, to fit in or because they notice that almost everyone else is drinking. For older adults, these social pressures may occur at restaurants or family events, when getting together with friends or in specific housing situations (e.g., retirement communities). There are several strategies to use when faced with this pressure. One possibility is to avoid these situations. This may be possible with casual acquaintances but becomes more challenging with close friends and family. In this case, the older adult should have strategies ready for times when they are offered a drink or feel social pressure to drink. It can be helpful to anticipate these situations in advance, such as when the client knows that a family event is coming up that involves drinking. If the client is trying to cut back, practitioners can work with the client to decide on how many drinks they will have at the event, and then practice how to respond if additional drinks are offered. There are many ways to do this. For example, if clients feel uncomfortable telling others that they are trying to control their drinking, they could say they are watching their weight, need to get up early the next day, or need to drive home and want to stay safe.

One consideration for drink refusal skills is that older adults may prefer to approach difficult interpersonal situations using passive coping strategies, such as doing nothing, keeping quiet, or changing the subject (Birditt et al., 2020). Because of this, older adults may not want to engage in drink refusal skills that are confrontational in nature. For example, one drink refusal strategy that can be taught in CBT is for the client to use the "broken record" technique where they simply repeat a similar phrase in response to offers to drink from a person pressuring them, such as "No, I'm not drinking." Another strategy is to be direct and not leave an opportunity to be asked later. For example, instead of saying, "Probably not, I have to get up early tomorrow," the client is encouraged to say, "No, I'm not drinking today." These approaches may feel too direct for older adults who may prefer to use more passive strategies. If drink refusal seems too difficult and a client wants to avoid drinking, it may be necessary to decline some high-risk social activities and seek out alternatives.

As with younger adults, some older clients use alcohol to manage negative emotional states, such as depression or anxiety. It can be helpful to provide mood management skills to older adults with unhealthy alcohol use, particularly if negative emotional states are identified as triggers. Cognitive restructuring can be used for mood management, with a focus on identifying unhelpful thoughts that contribute to negative moods instead of thoughts that contribute to alcohol use. This topic can be introduced by discussing with the client how negative moods are common among those with unhealthy alcohol use. The practitioner can further explain that negative moods can sometimes appear before alcohol use (emotional antecedent) and that, although drinking often leads to short-term improvement, alcohol use can lead to a worsening of mood after the initial effects have worn off. The client can be asked to consider if this pattern applies to them and how they experience mood as it relates to alcohol use. Following this, the practitioner can further emphasize the connection between situations, thoughts, and feelings, and how certain thoughts can lead to anxious or sad feelings. At this point, a thought record can be introduced that is specific to negative moods, as opposed to focusing on alcohol use. The thought record can be used to identify automatic thoughts that lead to negative mood states – for example, worrying excessively about the future or being overly self-critical. A similar process of cognitive restructuring can then occur where the client learns to challenge their own automatic thoughts and replace them with more realistic and balanced thoughts. Table 18 presents a summary of the components of CBT that are discussed in this chapter. Some of these treatment components are more appropriate for a higher-severity client who needs a longer-term treatment, such as managing thoughts about alcohol

Table 18. Cognitive and behavioral skills used in cognitive behavioral therapy (CBT) for unhealthy alcohol use

Session topic	Examples
Self-monitoring alcohol use	Introduce how tracking alcohol use can be helpful.
Identifying triggers for drinking	Assess all five domains for triggers: social, environmental, emotional, cognitive, and physical.
Increasing pleasant activities and behavioral activation	Use pleasant events scheduling to help the client engage in alternative activities besides alcohol use.
Enhancing social support networks	Assess the client's current social network and social opportunities. Practice specific skills during sessions, such as calling a friend to talk.
Managing thoughts about alcohol and drinking	Use thought records with the client to identify automatic thoughts that are associated with drinking and replace those thoughts with more balanced and realistic thoughts that are less likely to result in drinking.
Coping with cravings and urges to drink	Ask the client to write down urges to drink and what happened before and after the urge to drink.
Drink refusal skills	Assess the client's preferred refusal skills and practice during sessions.
Managing anxiety and depression	Use a thought record to track how automatic thoughts are related to negative mood states. Engage in cognitive restructuring with the client to replace automatic thoughts with more balanced and realistic thoughts that are less likely to result in negative moods.

and drinking and managing anxiety and depression, whereas others are appropriate for a brief intervention. This is because some of these skills may take longer to introduce, explain, model, and practice.

CBT with older clients can be delivered as individual or group treatment. One group treatment model developed for older adults is the Gerontology Alcohol Project (GAP; Center for Substance Abuse Treatment, 2005). This is a longer-term (16-session) treatment that is appropriate for clients who need a more intensive level of treatment. In this group treatment, clients work through nine modules after completing an assessment of alcohol use patterns and related problems. The modules are detailed in Table 19, and the content can be useful for practitioners to incorporate into group or individual CBT.

Table 19. Gerontology Alcohol Project treatment components

Treatment module	Session	Content
Analysis of alcohol behavior	Two sessions	Clients use the ABC model to determine antecedents, behaviors, and consequences of drinking
How to manage social pressure	Two sessions	Learn and practice drink refusal skills to use in high-risk social situations
How to manage situations at home and alone	One session	Skills for managing leisure time (pleasant events scheduling) and what to do when bored or lonely
How to manage negative thoughts and emotions associated with alcohol use	One or two sessions	Use cognitive restructuring to recognize negative self-talk and identify other ways to cope with negative emotions besides alcohol use
Managing anxiety and tension	Three sessions	Identifying anxiety and tensions as well as skills to reduce these emotions
Managing anger and frustration	Three sessions	The client learns to use assertiveness skills to manage anger, along with other techniques
Controlling alcohol use	One session	Recognize personal cues that often lead to alcohol use and skills to manage the cues
Coping with urges	Two sessions	Increase skills in recognizing that urges have a beginning and end period and that they become easier to resist once they are managed successfully
Preventing a slip from becoming a full return to drinking	One session	Use acquired behavioral and cognitive skills to manage slips

As an example of a specific technique used in GAP, Module 8 (coping with urges) has a helpful mnemonic to manage urges. The acronym is CRASH:

- Remember CONSEQUENCES of drinking and not drinking
- Get RID of alcoholic beverages and REMOVE yourself from the situation
- Engage in an incompatible ACTIVITY
- Use SKILLS to manage feelings
- Call for HELP if the urge persists

Clinical Vignette 3 demonstrates how CBT techniques can be introduced and used with older clients, following along with the client from the prior sections who sees sleep problems as a primary consequence of drinking.

> ### Clinical Vignette 3:
> ### Introducing CBT techniques to older clients
>
> **Practitioner:** Let's talk about your drinking patterns and your thoughts about alcohol. You said you drink in the evening with your partner. You mentioned that you often have a glass of wine or two at dinner, and then another glass or two of wine after dinner. Does that sound about right? (Introduce CBT Components about Drinking Patterns and Thoughts)
>
> **Client:** Yes, that's right.
>
> **Practitioner:** Let's talk about feelings or situations that seem connected with drinking. This can be useful in understanding drinking patterns and in thinking about how alcohol fits into your day overall. For example, what is your mood usually like before you have wine with dinner? (Emotional Antecedents)
>
> **Client:** Well by the end of the day, I am usually pretty tired. Like I said, my sleep has been really bad, and I am trying not to take naps during the day because that causes me even more sleep problems. So I feel tired. I guess you could say I'm a little cranky too, by the late afternoon.
>
> **Practitioner:** By dinner, you're feeling tired and a little cranky. What's going through your mind as you pour that glass of wine? (Behavioral and Cognitive Antecedents)
>
> **Client:** Well, that's a little hard to say since it's just kind of a habit. I don't really think too much about it before I drink. But I guess I might be thinking that having a glass of wine will help me feel more relaxed.
>
> **Practitioner:** It's a way to unwind. And maybe you are thinking that feeling relaxed will help you fall asleep later on? (Drinking Consequences)
>
> **Client:** Yeah, sleep could also be part of it. Drinking helps me feel less edgy. Like I said, I can be a little cranky at the end of the day. So the wine helps me unwind a little, relax.

Practitioner: This is great insight. What other things might help you relax? I wonder if there's anything you could do before dinner, so you aren't feeling quite on edge? (Managing Mood States)

Client: I like to walk around the neighborhood sometimes. I think I could start doing that again. I used to be more active during the day, but I guess I've been staying at home a lot more lately.

Practitioner: Tell me more about walking in the neighborhood. How has that been helpful? (Planning Alternative Activities and Behavioral Activation)

Client: Well, I usually feel better after I get some exercise. Physically I know it's good for me to be walking. I sometimes run into a few neighbors, and we chat a little. I like seeing my neighbors. And my wife will join me on the walk, and it's nice for us to have some time together.

Practitioner: There are a lot of things that you like about walking before dinner, even though lately you haven't been doing this as much. I wonder if you might be willing to try going for a walk before dinner a few times this week to see how it affects your mood. You can continue to track your thoughts and feelings in the thought record and we'll look it over next week. (Reinforcing Session Content and Thought Records)

6.7 Mutual Help Groups

Mutual help groups (MHGs) include 12-step programs such as Alcoholics Anonymous (AA) as well as other groups, including Self-Management and Recovery Training (SMART) Recovery, Moderation Management, LifeRing, Women for Sobriety, and Refuge Recovery, among others. The three most common alternatives to AA are SMART Recovery, LifeRing, and Women for Sobriety. This section primarily focuses on 12-step programs, with a brief overview of the other MHGs. One of the benefits of connecting clients to a 12-step program is that meetings are free, widely available in various geographic locations (rural, urban) and also at multiple times throughout the day as well as online. Providing additional opportunities for peer-to-peer support, such as through 12-step groups, can be a helpful addition to treatment for some clients.

Based on a recent systematic review of outcome studies, there is evidence that participation in 12-step programs such as AA is associated with improved long-term alcohol abstinence rates (Kelly et al., 2020). There are many ways in which individuals can participate in AA, and individuals can choose to be more or less involved. Some common ways to participate include attending meetings in person or online, working the steps, reading

12-step literature, doing service at the meetings (setting up, etc.), speaking at a meeting, calling other AA members for support, and identifying a sponsor, among others. AA participation can also help in expanding nondrinking social networks. Generally, each AA meeting has its own culture, and some meetings may be a better fit than others depending on the client's characteristics.

There is very little research on older adults' participation in 12-step programs for unhealthy alcohol use. In a qualitative study, Holland and colleagues (2016) found that adults aged 50 and older with a history of substance use were concerned about attending treatment group settings that included a wide age range of clients. This suggests that some 12-step programs may not be seen as a good fit by older adults because of the heterogeneity of group members' ages. However, when older adults do attend 12-step programs, they appear to benefit from participation. In a 20-year study of adults aged 55 to 65 with unhealthy alcohol use, obtaining help from 12-step programs was associated with improved alcohol outcomes at 10- and 20-year follow-ups (Moos et al., 2010). For older adults who have never attended MHGs, practitioners may need to follow up more frequently to check in with the client about meeting fit and troubleshoot any concerns that clients report about meeting format or content.

Although many practitioners recommend that clients attend 12-step programs, some clients do not follow through on the recommendation to attend AA. There are several possible reasons for this. Some clients may not feel comfortable with aspects of the AA philosophy (e.g., having to admit powerlessness over alcohol, reliance on a higher power) or with attending a meeting on their own where they may not know anyone. To address these concerns, there are both formal and informal ways that practitioners can facilitate older clients' involvement in AA. For example, 12-step facilitation therapy (TSF) is a structured intervention focused on getting clients connected to 12-step programs (Kelly & McCrady, 2008). TSF typically consists of four to 12 sessions of individual or group treatment. The content of TSF sessions includes exploring different 12-step themes such as powerlessness, spirituality, and personal responsibility, exploring the client's attitudes about those themes and other components of 12-step support groups, and identifying barriers that limit client willingness to participate. It should be noted that some sessions of the TSF treatment manual are more confrontational in nature and need to be adapted for older adults, who tend to respond better to less confrontational approaches (SAMHSA, 2020). For example, the TSF manual suggests discussion of denial and arrogance, which are listed as common personality traits of individuals with unhealthy alcohol use. This has the potential to alienate older clients and reinforce negative stereotypes surrounding unhealthy alcohol use. Instead, the practitioner can keep the discussion focused on alcohol-related problems that the client has identified.

Other programs similar to TSF have a shorter format and are group-based. For example, Making Alcoholics Anonymous Easier (MAAEZ; Kaskutas et al., 2009) is a group treatment that focuses on how to choose meetings; the benefits of AA on long-term success in reducing alcohol use; different ways to think about the spirituality component of AA; myths, etiquette, and rules for AA; and the process of selecting a sponsor. To date there have not been any studies of TSF among older adults.

Although practitioners may not wish to formally use a group-based 12-step facilitation protocol, some components may be helpful when trying to connect an older client to AA. For example, practitioners can explore the beliefs that clients have about AA, both positive and negative. Practitioners can also discuss the typical rules of an AA meeting so that clients attending for the first time know what to expect. An additional suggestion for practitioners includes contacting a local AA meeting together with a client on the phone and asking for a peer to accompany their client to their first meeting.

An important aspect of 12-step facilitation includes addressing possible concerns about the spirituality component of AA. Sometimes clients are reluctant to attend AA because their conception of AA is that you have to believe in "a power greater than yourself." Although there are options for MHGs that are not spiritual (see below), the spirituality component in AA can often be interpreted more broadly than standard conceptions of God or familiar religions. For example, the AA group itself can be considered the higher power, or it might be ideas about nature, the universe, love, or another spiritual power that resonates with the client.

There are options for older clients who do not want to attend AA, though evaluations of non-12-step MHGs for older adults are limited. Almost all MHGs encourage participants to work toward abstinence with the exception of Moderation Management. Moderation Management encourages an initial 1-month period of sobriety, followed by a personal decision to maintain abstinence or consume alcohol in moderation. As noted earlier in this chapter, harm reduction approaches may be a better fit for older adults; Moderation Management may be worth discussing with clients to decide if it is a good fit for them.

SMART Recovery is a secular group that is modeled on CBT and focuses on four main components, including increasing and maintaining motivation; managing urges and cravings; managing emotions, thoughts, and behaviors; and finding balance in life. SMART Recovery focuses on evidence-based strategies that are self-empowering and can be implemented by a nonprofessional volunteer. Whereas traditional 12-step groups focus more on an external locus of control (i.e., giving up power), SMART Recovery emphasizes an internal locus of control, such as by members learning new techniques and skills to manage unhealthy alcohol use (Horvath & Yeterian, 2012).

LifeRing identifies as a secular group that encourages participants to find control within themselves by focusing on the *addict self* and the *sober self*, with a goal of strengthening the sober self. The underlying philosophy focuses on the 3-S approach: *sobriety*, *secularity*, and *self-help*. Abstinence is encouraged, and there is no specific discussion of spirituality during meetings. Meetings focus on strengthening each individual's own motivation to stay sober, as opposed to a focus on group support.

Women for Sobriety aims to help women change thoughts and behaviors related to substance use with a focus on five values: compassion, connection, empowerment, love, and respect. Specific strategies used in Women for Sobriety include positive reinforcement through approval and encouragement toward sobriety, cognitive strategies such as increasing positive thinking, relaxation techniques, and group involvement.

Finally, Refuge Recovery takes a Buddhist and mindfulness-based approach to recovery. Their philosophy focuses on the Four Noble Truths and the Eightfold Path from the Buddhist philosophy.

If you are seeing an older adult who has never attended a MHG, it may be helpful to review and discuss all the options, including the groups described in this section that are not based on 12-step programs. Some of these options may be less available in rural areas and may have fewer meeting times, such that they are not as accessible as AA, but a growing number have meetings and content online.

6.8   Family-Involved Treatments

Interventions that include family members can be very useful for some clients. *Alcohol-focused behavioral couples therapy* (ABCT) is an evidence-based CBT treatment (see McCrady et al. 2016). This model of treatment proposes reciprocal relationships between alcohol (and other substance use) and interpersonal relationship functioning. Thus, targeting the client's drinking, improved coping skills for both partners, and the relationship is key to achieving and maintaining changes in drinking. ABCT includes activities focused on the client's drinking, such as self-monitoring of cravings for alcohol and drinking behaviors (e.g., quantity and frequency, time of day), an analysis of the chain of events that lead to drinking (e.g., a functional analysis of drinking), and coping skills for alcohol-related cravings and life stressors. Relational targets of treatment include communication skills, problemsolving skills, increasing shared positive activities, and increasing awareness of the partner's positive behaviors (e.g., nondrinking behaviors and other behaviors viewed as positive, such as taking care of a household chore). ABCT results in reduced drinking, reduced intimate partner violence, and improvements in overall relationship quality. ABCT may be particularly helpful in older adult couples where drinking has been a long-standing pattern. In these instances, both partners may be inadvertently contributing to sustained and maladaptive coping patterns in the relationship.

The *community reinforcement and family training* (CRAFT) approach is designed for the family members of individuals with substance use disorders and is an option for the family members of older adults looking for tools to support their loved one with unhealthy alcohol use (Roozen et al., 2010). CRAFT is offered as individual or group therapy and also via self-help resources. CRAFT teaches family members strategies to engage their loved one in treatment (if their family member is resistant to treatment), effective communication strategies, how to positively reinforce abstinence, how to respond when their loved one is drinking heavily, and how to encourage the loved one's retention in treatment for unhealthy alcohol use. CRAFT may have particular applications for family members, (e.g., partner, adult children, siblings) seeking strategies to their loved one's recovery, given the potentially complex family dynamics of assisting a parent or other older relative.

6.9 Effectiveness of Treatments for Unhealthy Alcohol Use Among Older Adults

This section will first review the effectiveness of alcohol treatments among older adults versus other age groups, including both short-term and long-term treatment studies. Following this, there is a review of outcome data among older adults for interventions discussed in this chapter. Many of the described treatments and MHGs have been used with older clients but lack evidence from randomized controlled trials, which is a major limitation in this area of research and clinical practice. Additionally, there is a paucity of recent studies evaluating treatments with older adults; however, many earlier studies are consistent with current recommendations around the use of CBT for older adults with unhealthy alcohol use (SAMHSA, 2020).

It is unclear if older adults with unhealthy alcohol use have better or worse treatment results than other age groups, regardless of the specific treatment intervention. In a study of 1-month outcomes following residential substance use treatment, Oslin and colleagues (2005) found that older adults entered treatment with more health problems and less outpatient treatment experience, along with lower severity of alcohol use. At 1-month follow-up, older adults were less likely to have contacted a sponsor or attended formal outpatient aftercare compared with middle-aged adults. In this study, older adults were also less likely to report that their quality of life was much or somewhat improved after treatment.

In a 6-month study of an outpatient alcohol and drug treatment program, researchers compared clients aged 55 and over to those 40–54 and 18–40 (Satre et al., 2003). Components of treatment included supportive group therapy, psychoeducation, behavioral relapse prevention, and family-oriented therapy. Participants attended 12-step meetings off-site. At 6 months, 55% of adults aged 55 and over reported abstinence from both alcohol and drugs, versus 59% of adults aged 40–54, and 50% of adults aged 18–40, indicating no significant difference in outcomes by age.

Older adults may have more support consistent with treatment efforts compared with younger adults. In a 5-year study, Satre and colleagues (2004) found that older adults reported having fewer friends who encouraged alcohol use compared with younger adults, though were less likely to have ever considered themselves a member of a 12-step program. At a 5-year follow-up, older adults had higher 30-day and past-year abstinence rates compared with younger adults. When all variables were considered together in one analysis, age was not a significant predictor of outcomes. Significant predictors that emerged were longer treatment retention and not having friends who encouraged alcohol use. These results suggest that older adults may have protective factors that lead to better outcomes, such as staying longer in treatment and having fewer individuals in their social network who might actively interfere in their recovery.

Focusing on specific treatments, there is some support for the use of MI in behavior change interventions among older adults, based on limited research (Cummings et al., 2009). Almost all of this work examines brief interventions that use a MI approach in primary care, as outlined in the following paragraphs on results of randomized controlled trials. For example, in a comparison of younger and older adults completing a brief intervention in primary care, Gordon and colleagues (2003) found that three intervention approaches (MI, brief advice, and usual care) resulted in similar outcomes (i.e., number of days abstained, number of drinks per day, and days in the past month when alcohol was consumed), and both older and younger adults had similar reductions in outcomes at 1-year follow-up.

Few randomized controlled trials have evaluated treatments among older adults with unhealthy alcohol use. Rather, treatments tested on younger and middle-aged adults are extended to use with older adults with some content and format adaptations. Exceptions include randomized controlled trials conducted on brief intervention models used in primary care for older adults with unhealthy alcohol use. Some of these include Project Guiding Older

Adult Lifestyles (Project GOAL; Fleming et al., 1999), Healthy Living as You Age (Moore et al., 2011), Project Senior Health and Alcohol Risk Education (Project SHARE; Ettner et al., 2014), and the Florida Brief Intervention and Treatment for Elders (BRITE) project (Schonfeld et al., 2010). Relevant outcome data are provided below, though these treatments are often implemented with the assistance of an interdisciplinary team, which may not be available to some practitioners. Nevertheless, the content of the brief intervention could be helpful for practitioners looking to implement a short-term treatment with an older client who has low-severity unhealthy alcohol use.

Project GOAL involves a 30-minute assessment session for older adults who screen positive for drinking above recommended limits. Following the assessment session, participants receive either a health workbook (control group) or the workbook plus two short (10-15 minute) sessions with their physician. During the sessions with the physician, an alcohol consumption agreement is created and given to the client in the form of a prescription. The Project GOAL intervention reduced alcohol use in the past week, episodes of binge drinking, and the frequency of excessive drinking at 3, 6, and 12 months postintervention (Fleming et al., 1999).

In a study of the Healthy Living as You Age program, participants aged 55 and over were screened by phone to identify patterns of unhealthy alcohol use, based on quantity and frequency of drinking, health risk factors, and alcohol-related problems (Moore et al., 2011). In a controlled trial, participants received either a booklet on health behaviors (control) or personalized feedback on health behaviors plus a drinking diary and three telephone counseling sessions using MI techniques from a health educator (active intervention condition). At 3-month follow-up, participants in the intervention condition reported lower rates of unhealthy alcohol use. At 12-month follow-up, outcomes were mixed. Unhealthy alcohol use did not differ between the two groups, although intervention participants reported fewer drinks consumed in the prior week.

Project SHARE was conducted in primary care settings (Ettner et al., 2014). The intervention included personalized reports, educational materials, drinking diaries, physician advice during office visits, and telephone counseling delivered by a health educator. The control group received treatment as usual, which may or may not have included feedback on their drinking. In addition to the treatment components described in this section, participants in the intervention group also received three phone calls from a health educator. During these calls, the health educator answered questions about the written materials and engaged in the following five steps: (a) assessment and direct feedback, (b) negotiation and goal setting, (c) behavioral modification techniques, (d) self-help-directed bibliotherapy, and (e) follow-up and reinforcement. At the follow-up assessments, both groups decreased alcohol consumption, though the intervention group had a larger decrease compared with the control group. For example, at 6-month follow-up, rates of unhealthy alcohol use were 60 % in the intervention group and 72 % in the control groups. Rates of unhealthy alcohol use decreased further at 12-month follow-up to 56 % in the intervention group and 67 % in the control group.

In another study of a MI-based brief intervention in medical and social services settings, the BRITE project (Schonfeld et al., 2010) followed the SBIRT model and offered a brief intervention to older adults who screened positive for unhealthy alcohol use. This intervention typically occurred outside of primary care in order to screen individuals in social services settings, such as senior centers. Upon screening positive, the brief intervention consisted of one to five sessions, often provided in the participant's home and primarily focused on goal setting, consequences of drinking, and reasons for wanting to cut back. Those who received the brief intervention showed improvement in alcohol use at 1-month follow-up (Schonfeld, et al., 2010). The studies reviewed regarding brief MI-based interventions in primary care (Fleming et al., 1999; Ettner et al., 2014; Moore et al., 2011; Schonfeld et al., 2010) highlight the positive impact of using brief MI-based interventions for individuals with lower-severity alcohol use.

CBT-based interventions for unhealthy alcohol use among older adults have shown improvements in abstinence rates but have not been tested in comparison with a control group. For example, in a study examining age differences in response to extended CBT (16 sessions), a relationship enhancement intervention consisting of six sessions of CBT, eight sessions with a partner, and two group sessions, or vocational and relationship enhancement (six sessions of CBT, four partner sessions, and four vocational sessions), Rice and colleagues (1993) found that all three treatments performed equally well among younger adults (18–29 years old). Middle-aged adults (30–49 years old) had better outcomes in the relationship enhancement condition and older adults (50 years and older) had better outcomes in the CBT-only condition. In this study, the primary outcomes were percentage of days abstinent and percentage of heavy drinking days in the past 3 months.

Studies on CBT-based treatments for older adults have focused on adaptations of the Gerontology Alcohol Project (GAP), a 16-session CBT-based group treatment. The GAP intervention consists of an assessment of alcohol use, followed by nine modules of CBT (e.g., analysis of alcohol use behavior). Although evaluations of GAP examined participants' posttreatment drinking outcomes, none of the studies used a control group. In a study of GAP treatment among older adults aged 55 and over with unhealthy alcohol use, 74 % of participants achieved their self-selected goal of abstinence or low-risk drinking at 1-year follow-up (Dupree et al., 1984). In another examination of outcomes of CBT-based treatment using the GAP model, Schonfeld and colleagues (2000) followed older adult participants (60 years and older) for 6 months after completing a CBT-based group treatment program. Of 110 participants, 45 % completed at least 13 of the 16 CBT sessions. Those who completed treatment were significantly more likely to be abstinent at 6-month follow-up compared with those who did not complete the treatment. Although the outcome data for CBT-based treatments among older adults with unhealthy alcohol use is dated and from uncontrolled trials, the most recent SAMHSA TIP for substance use problems in older adults (SAMHSA, 2020) recommends CBT as a primary treatment for older clients due its large literature base both with other age groups and with older adults for other mental health conditions.

There is some research to suggest that older adults are less likely to engage in MHGs such as 12-step programs, though almost all of this research is observational or qualitative. For example, Holland and colleagues (2016) found that, in a qualitative study of treatment preferences of older adults seeking substance use treatment, participants reported that their treatment success was limited by having participants of multiple ages in the group instead of a group specific to older adults. In a 20-year study of adults aged 55 to 65 with unhealthy alcohol use, obtaining help from 12-step programs was associated with a lower likelihood of high-risk alcohol consumption (above recommended guidelines) and was also associated with fewer problems resulting from drinking at 10- and 20-year follow-ups (Moos et al., 2010). In contrast, obtaining help from family, friends, and from professional sources was not significantly associated with outcomes, suggesting that there was a unique benefit of AA for these participants. Therefore, older adults appear to benefit from MHGs even if they are less likely to attend compared with other age groups.

Based on this limited evidence, it appears that older adults benefit as much from alcohol use treatment as, or more than, other age groups. All of the treatments reviewed so far are evidence-based treatments and have significant support for their use in general adult populations. Although these interventions may work well with individual clients depending on their circumstances, caution is needed in applying treatments that have not been examined specifically for use with older adults. For example, practitioners may find that some components of treatment (e.g., high-risk situations and coping skills) do not adapt well to older adults, who are typically facing different life stressors than other age groups.

6.10 Conclusions: Psychological Interventions for Unhealthy Alcohol Use

Although there are many psychological treatments available for unhealthy alcohol use, many of them have not been studied among older adults. Brief interventions, MI, and CBT are the most common interventions for unhealthy alcohol use and also have the most support for use with older adults. Family-involved treatments may also be appropriate for older couples. Some treatment adaptations may be needed for older adults, to better tailor treatment to their specific situation. Starting with the least restrictive option, practitioners might first consider referral to a MHG along with a brief intervention focused on MI and specific skills from a CBT treatment protocol. Although outcome data are limited for older adults, older adults appear to benefit from treatment as much as other age groups.

7
Pharmacological Interventions

Although the focus of this book is primarily on psychological interventions, practitioners should be aware of medications that can help clients reduce drinking or achieve abstinence. The majority of clients will likely not need medication for unhealthy alcohol use; however, clients may have questions about these medications or may have previously had a prescription for one of the common medications for alcohol use disorder (AUD), depending on the treatment setting. There are three primary medications approved by the US Food and Drug Administration for AUD: disulfiram, naltrexone (oral and injectable), and acamprosate. There are pros and cons for use of each medication among older adults. The addition of AUD medications to treatment increases the likelihood of drug–drug interactions, which may be a concern for medically complex older adults who are on multiple prescription medications. There have been few clinical trials for these medications that included older adults.

7.1   Disulfiram

Disulfiram (Antabuse) is considered a deterrent agent. If alcohol is consumed while on disulfiram, unpleasant effects will typically occur within 10 minutes and can last for up to an hour. These side effects include nausea, headache, vomiting, face flush, and chest pain, among others. The medication is taken orally once a day. Individuals should not have had any alcohol for 12 hrs prior to their first dose. Disulfiram is generally not recommended for older adults because of the possibility of severe side effects. For example, if an older person consumed alcohol while on disulfiram, and they were living alone, there could be safety concerns if they started experiencing the unpleasant effects of disulfiram (vomiting, etc.), which may be more likely to lead to dehydration among older adults compared with other age groups. Disulfiram is also contraindicated among individuals who have a history of seizures, cerebrovascular disease, or peripheral neuropathy. The last two conditions may be present in medically complex older adults. Disulfiram can also interact with medications used to treat bacterial infections, such as cephalosporins, chloramphenicol, ketoconazole, and metronidazole (Caputo et al., 2012).

7.2 Naltrexone

Naltrexone is an antagonist that blocks the effects of alcohol and therefore makes alcohol less reinforcing. This may lead to fewer cravings. Naltrexone can be taken either as a tablet or as an injectable. For those taking tablets, it is common to start with a dose of 50 mg once per day. Some older adults may prefer the injectable form to reduce the number of daily medications they need to take as pills. The injectable form of the drug is called Vivitrol. Vivitrol is given intramuscularly at 380 mg once per month. It is safe for long-term use. Naltrexone is metabolized in the liver. In large doses, naltrexone can cause liver toxicity, though this is uncommon if the client is taking a recommended dose. Because of the possibility of liver toxicity, naltrexone is contraindicated in clients with liver dysfunction, such as hepatitis or cirrhosis. Naltrexone may also be problematic for older adults who are prescribed opiate-based analgesics for pain. The mechanism of action for naltrexone is that it blocks the effects of opioids, so this could lead to lower effectiveness of pain medications.

There are limited studies on the use of naltrexone among older adults. A systematic review by Tampi and colleagues (2019) identified two double-blind randomized controlled trials of naltrexone among older adults. There were no studies identified that assessed the use of disulfiram or acamprosate among older adults. In one of the studies included in the Tampi and colleagues (2019) article, Oslin and colleagues (1997) found that there were no significant differences in abstinence rates between the two groups (naltrexone vs. placebo), and there were no significant differences in adverse effects between treatment groups. In both groups, sleep disturbances and anxiety were the most commonly reported adverse effects. In a second study, Oslin and colleagues (2005) tested the combination of naltrexone and sertraline (Zoloft) for older adults who met criteria for both AUD and depression. Results indicated that return to alcohol use was not significantly different between the naltrexone group (35%) and the placebo group (32%). Abstinence rates were also not significantly different between the naltrexone group (43%) and the placebo group (54%), which the authors hypothesized was related to individual differences in the effect of naltrexone on neurotransmission.

7.3 Acamprosate

Acamprosate reduces cravings for alcohol, though the specific mechanism is unclear. Acamprosate is metabolized in the kidneys and therefore could be an alternative to naltrexone for older adults who have liver dysfunction. That being said, there are no randomized controlled trials of acamprosate among older adults. Acamprosate is contraindicated in clients with kidney problems. Acamprosate is usually taken three times per day. This is in contrast to once-a-day oral dosing or a monthly injection for naltrexone. Therefore, acamprosate may not be a good choice for older adults, since the need for more frequent dosing increases the likelihood of mistakes in taking the medication.

7.4 Integrating Pharmacotherapy With Psychotherapy

There are different ways in which AUD medications can be incorporated into behavioral treatments. For example, Oslin and colleagues (2002) examined the combination of motivational interviewing (MI) sessions with naltrexone. Participants attended MI-consistent nonconfrontational sessions that focused on motivating participants to change and treatment adherence. Older adults were more adherent to naltrexone and attended more therapy sessions compared with younger adults. This study suggests that providing MI-consistent psychotherapy in combination with naltrexone to older adults can lead to improved engagement in both treatments. For practitioners in independent practice, treatment integration may involve helping the client develop a plan to adhere to their naltrexone treatment regimen, or using psychotherapy to focus on the client's other goals in relation to unhealthy alcohol use.

Building on cognitive behavioral therapy (CBT) or MI approaches, practitioners can frame taking medications as a useful behavior in supporting alcohol use reduction. Practitioners may also assist older clients in developing a plan to adhere to medications, such as planning for when clients will take the medication or by involving supportive family members if needed. Practitioners could also use some of the techniques described in Section 6.6 on CBT to better understand triggers for unhealthy alcohol use and work to reduce or avoid those triggers while using AUD medication as a way of making overall treatment more effective.

7.5 Conclusions: Pharmacological Interventions

The studies reviewed in this section suggest that naltrexone may be an option for older adults with alcohol dependence if it is medically appropriate. Older adults should discuss these medication options with their physicians, though it can be helpful for mental health practitioners to be informed about primary medication options for AUDs, including potential concerns and contraindications for older adults.

8
Cultural Adaptations

Few studies have examined how race, culture, gender, and sexual and gender minority status influence treatment outcomes among older adults with unhealthy alcohol use. Although some studies focus on how prevalence rates of unhealthy alcohol use differ among older adults from minority groups in the US (see Section 2.2 Prevalence of Unhealthy Alcohol Use Among Older Adults), this line of research does not extend to treatment outcomes. Given the lack of research on substance use treatment outcomes by race and culture among older adults, this chapter reviews cultural adaptations for treatments that can be used across all adult age groups. Also included is a discussion of unhealthy alcohol use among older women compared with older men, including implications for treatment.

8.1   Cultural Adaptations to Treatment

There is a growing amount of research on cultural adaptations of *screening, brief intervention, and referral to treatment* (SBIRT) and motivational interviewing (MI) for unhealthy alcohol use (Green, 2018; Ornelas et al., 2015). Generally, *cultural adaptation* refers to modifying an existing evidence-based treatment to consider language, culture, and context (Bernal et al., 2009). There are many theoretical frameworks available to guide cultural adaptations. For example, the *ecological validity model* examines eight dimensions of how interventions can be adapted, including language, persons, metaphors, content, concepts, goals, methods, and context (Bernal et al., 2009). Other frameworks for cultural adaptation focus on surface versus deep adaptations. *Surface adaptations* refer to modification of intervention materials or messages to fit within a specific culture. *Deep adaptations* refer to incorporation of how the culture explains the cause, course, and treatment of the target behavior. Although this research has not included older adults, some themes can be applied to working with older adults from racial and ethnic minority populations.

Starting with screening and assessment, several measures have been validated on diverse populations and are translated for use with non-English speakers. For instance, the full 10-item Alcohol Use Disorders Identification Test (AUDIT) was validated on individuals identifying as Black, Latinx/Hispanic, and Northern Plains American Indians (Burrow-Sánchez &

Nielsen, 2020). The full AUDIT is available in Arabic, Korean, and five Chinese languages. The AUDIT-C is also available in multiple languages (e.g., Arabic, Spanish, Korean), and validity studies have included multiple racial and ethnicity minority groups. Other screening measures have been translated or evaluated in diverse populations (see Manuel et al., 2015, for a review).

A number of studies have examined cultural adaptations to brief treatments for unhealthy alcohol use, including SBIRT and MI. Lee and colleagues (2019) conducted a trial of MI adapted for use with Latinx individuals with unhealthy alcohol use. In this study, MI was adapted for Spanish and English-speaking Latinx drinkers and included components specific to the needs of this population, including stress related to US immigration, ethnic-specific drinking norms, and factors such as discrimination, acculturation stress, and social isolation. Culturally adapted MI was compared with standard MI (both delivered in a single session). Participants in both conditions reported improvements in drinking (as measured by percentage of heavy drinking days and frequency of negative consequences), with no differences between treatment conditions. Culturally adapted MI resulted in improvement in some outcomes compared with standard MI, such as frequency of negative consequences among participants who reported lower levels of acculturation and higher levels of discrimination.

In a review of cultural adaptations of MI for various health behaviors, including unhealthy alcohol use, Self and colleagues (2022) found that the majority of studies on adaptations were focused on Latinx or Black populations. Among studies that included a control condition ($n = 17$), 10 studies found that the cultural adaptation condition was favored over the MI control condition when examining the primary outcome measure. The most commonly adapted elements from the Bernal and colleagues (2009) framework included content, context, and concepts.

In a cultural adaptation of SBIRT among Latinx day laborers, Ornelas and colleagues (2015) found in qualitative interviews that Latinx day laborers used alcohol to relieve stress related to immigration, such as feeling lonely or guilty about being away from their families. Alcohol was also used to relieve depression and anxiety. Many reported that unhealthy alcohol use was seen as acceptable among other Latinx individuals in their community. The participants preferred to receive interventions in Spanish from a provider who could relate to their culture. Lack of cultural sensitivity was often cited as a barrier to services. There was also concern about seeking public services for those who were undocumented. Participants reported dissatisfaction with existing services such as 12-step groups, partially because few were available in Spanish. Based on these results, the authors suggested that potential cultural adaptations to SBIRT for this population include services in

Spanish, incorporating the social and cultural context of men, and providing services at a convenient location and at a low cost.

These recommendations are consistent with a review of cultural adaptations to SBIRT by Burrow-Sánchez and Nielsen (2020), which suggests that cultural adaptations to SBIRT focus on use of screening instruments that are appropriate for the population, use of strategies that are culturally relevant and sensitive to the specific population, and increasing cultural competence to work with racially and ethnically diverse populations, as well as considering the importance of the therapeutic relationship. The authors emphasize that lack of a positive therapeutic relationship will significantly reduce the effectiveness of any cultural adaptations offered in treatment. Building on this, Satre and colleagues (2015) reviewed guidelines for cultural adaptations of SBIRT and MI, as presented in Table 20.

8.2 Treatment Considerations for Sexual and Gender Minority Older Adults

Older sexual and gender minority adults have a higher likelihood of unhealthy alcohol use compared with heterosexual older adults (Han et al., 2020). The higher prevalence rates may be related to the chronic stress of historical and current discrimination against those identifying as sexual and gender minorities (Goldhammer et al., 2019). Although there are no published treatment adaptations for unhealthy alcohol use among sexual and gender minority older adults, Goldhammer and colleagues (2019) offers guidelines to meet their behavioral health needs. Treatment considerations focus on an inclusive clinical environment and providing affirming clinical care. Goldhammer and colleagues (2019) suggest that an inclusive clinical environment includes lesbian, gay, bisexual, and transgender (LGBT)-inclusive policies, training for staff in LGBT care, materials that portray gender-diverse individuals, and collection of data on sexual orientation and gender identity, with an option to not answer if that is preferred. Affirming clinical care includes assessment of minority stress; validation and recognition of identity, relationships, and families of choice; integrated behavioral health care to ensure that services are easy to access; and promotion of social and community connectedness. In the model proposed by Goldhammer and colleagues (2019), an inclusive clinical environment and provision of affirming clinical care should work to address and reduce the adverse health effects experienced by sexual and gender minority older adults.

8 Cultural Adaptations 85

Table 20. Culturally competent SBIRT and MI guidelines. Adapted from Satre and colleagues (2015).

Guideline	Clinical application
Implement skills that are fundamental to successful cross-cultural encounters, including empathy, curiosity, and respect.	Engage in active listening and support clients' own decision making, consistent with core SBIRT and MI approaches.
Seek out knowledge about racial and ethnic minority populations.	Individual assessment of client's experiences and values will aid in avoiding stereotyping.
Understand the meaning of illness for each client.	Assess client's goals based on their view of illness.
Focus on social context and social support.	Practitioners can ask about the client's environment, finances, social stressors, immigration, and social networks.
Assess client's language preference.	Translate materials as needed, employ multilingual staff, and use screening instruments that are validated on racial and ethnic minority groups.
Provide appropriate education based on the client's health literacy levels.	Assess the client's health literacy level and provide MI-consistent health information on alcohol use that is at the client's level.
When implementing cross-cultural interventions, incorporate members of the community.	For some racial and ethnic minority groups, treatment for unhealthy alcohol use may be more acceptable when community members assist in organizing treatment.
Consider a family-centered approach.	Assess the impact of alcohol use on the family and explore the family context.
When appropriate, integrate traditional spirituality and traditional cultural practices.	Incorporation of traditional cultural practices may have positive effects on alcohol use.
Negotiate mutually agreeable treatment options.	Alcohol treatment should be based on the client's preferences and their unique context.

Note. MI = motivational interviewing; SBIRT = screening, brief intervention, and referral to treatment.

8.3 Treatment Considerations for Older Women

Older women who engage in unhealthy alcohol use may have additional challenges for treatment, including social isolation and guilt around alcohol use (Epstein et al., 2007; Han et al., 2017). For older women, it can be particularly hard to cut back if they have a spouse or partner with unhealthy alcohol use. Barriers to treatment for older women also include increased stigma surrounding drinking and treatment for unhealthy alcohol use (Epstein et al., 2007). Although not specific to older adults, women with unhealthy alcohol use are more likely to have comorbid mental health disorders, as compared with men. For instance, women with alcohol use disorder (AUD) experience higher rates of comorbid depression and anxiety than men with AUD (for a review, see Peltier et al., 2019). Women tend to have more prescriptions than men, increasing the risk of prescription misuse and also the risk of alcohol–medication interactions. Women with unhealthy alcohol use are also more likely to have social support networks that include those with unhealthy alcohol use and those who do not support recovery (Epstein, McCrady, Hallgren, Cook, et al., 2018).

Research by Satre and colleagues examined differences in outcomes for treatment of unhealthy alcohol use between older men and women. In a study of 6-month outcomes of older men and women (aged 55+) in an outpatient addictions program, Satre, Mertens, and Weisner (2004) found that women initiated heavy drinking at a later age than men but had similar drinking levels at intake. At follow-up, 79 % of women reported abstinence in the past 30 days, compared with 54 % of men. Among those who were still using alcohol, older men reported more frequent instances of unhealthy alcohol use compared with older women. Similar results were found when examining gender differences in 5-year outcomes among older adults (aged 55+) completing a chemical dependency program (Satre, Mertens, Areán, & Weisner, 2004). At 5-year follow-up, older women were more likely to be abstinent than older men. Within groups, age was significant for women only; older women were more likely to be abstinent than younger women, but this difference was not seen among men (younger and older men had similar abstinence rates). Older women were also more likely to stay in treatment than older men (mean 21 weeks vs. 10 weeks).

Women-specific treatments have been developed to address the unique needs of this population. As mentioned in Section 6.7 Mutual Help Groups, Women for Sobriety is a mutual help group (MHG) focused on the specific needs of women with unhealthy alcohol use. Women for Sobriety focuses on women's strengths, and women are asked to introduce themselves by saying their name and "I am a competent woman." In a longitudinal study comparing AA with LifeRing, SMART Recovery, and Women for Sobriety, Zemore and colleagues (2018) found that primary group affiliation was not associated with the outcome of alcohol-related problems at 1-year follow-up. This suggests that Women for Sobriety is as effective as other MHGs and should be offered as an option to older women.

Epstein and colleagues have developed a female-specific cognitive behavioral therapy (FS-CBT) for women with unhealthy alcohol use (Epstein, McCrady, Hallgren, Cook, et al., 2018). This 12-session treatment approach includes themes such as self-care and self-confidence, interpersonal functioning, and ways to increase social support. The treatment content is delivered using women-specific language, examples, illustrations, and worksheets. A trial of FS-CBT versus gender-neutral CBT demonstrated that women in both conditions were highly engaged and satisfied with treatment. Additionally, women in both conditions reported significant reductions in drinking. This study, although not focused exclusively on older women (average age was 48 years), offers an evidence-based alternative for women who prefer female-specific treatment options.

A later trial evaluated the efficacy of 12 sessions of FS-CBT delivered as a group treatment (G-FS-CBT) versus individual female-specific CBT. Again, women in both conditions were highly satisfied with treatment and reported similar improvements in drinking outcomes (Epstein, McCrady, Hallgren, Gaba, et al., 2018). These approaches may be particularly beneficial to older adult women, who may be more reluctant to engage in treatment for unhealthy alcohol use.

Taken together with the information in Section 2.2 Prevalence of Unhealthy Alcohol Use Among Older Adults, older women are emerging as a group of concern for unhealthy alcohol use, and treatment modifications may be beneficial. For example, treatment might be adapted to include a specific focus on interpersonal and emotional triggers for drinking, increasing social support for abstinence, enhancing healthy relationships, and enhancing a sense of self and personal agency, as well as treatment of comorbid internalizing disorders (Epstein, McCrady, Hallgren, Cook, et al., 2018).

8.4 Conclusions: Cultural Adaptations

Although research is very limited on cultural adaptations for older adults with unhealthy alcohol use, it is beneficial to consider the evidence for cultural adaptations and whether similar adaptations may be effective for some older clients. For racial and ethnic minority older adults, this may include the role of acculturation and discrimination in the context of unhealthy alcohol use, in addition to adaptation of materials into a preferred language. For gender and sexual minority older adults, this includes consideration of how to provide an inclusive clinical environment and affirming clinical care in the context of unhealthy alcohol use. Finally, older women may benefit from adaptations that have a different focus than gender-neutral treatments – for example, those focusing on interpersonal triggers and social support networks supportive of recovery.

9
General Conclusions

In light of the increasing number of older adults in the US, practitioners may find themselves working with older adult clients more frequently. This book highlights that unhealthy alcohol use among older adults is underdiagnosed and undertreated, and that there are few treatments designed specifically for older adults with unhealthy alcohol use. At the same time, unhealthy alcohol use is on the rise among older adults, specifically among certain groups. It is not uncommon for unhealthy alcohol use to be detected among older adults only when significant consequences occur, such as falls, car accidents, or neglect. There are also lifespan developmental factors to consider when working with older adults with unhealthy alcohol use, including generational views on alcohol and substance use, as well as changes over the lifespan that may increase the risk for unhealthy alcohol use, such as retirement and other transitions. Additionally, there are modifications to treatment that may be needed for some older adult clients, such as pacing of the material and the need for visual, hearing, cognitive, or other accommodations.

One primary recommendation from this book is that practitioners should screen all older adult clients for alcohol use, even long-term clients that have not previously indicated a problem with alcohol. When assessing unhealthy alcohol use among older adults, consider life transitions that may increase alcohol use, and health problems or medications that may interact with alcohol use. Brief interventions should be considered first, in line with the screening, brief intervention, and referral to treatment (SBIRT) model. Brief interventions may work well for the majority of clients. For those needing more treatment, cognitive behavioral therapy (CBT) and motivational interviewing (MI) are empirically supported, though research is limited on randomized controlled trials of treatments for unhealthy alcohol use that include older adults. Treatment adaptations that apply specifically to older adults include coordinating care with other health care providers, considering a harm reduction rather than an abstinence approach, slowing the pace of treatment for older adults with cognitive impairments, using a nonconfrontational treatment approach, and considering the unique contexts and treatment adaptations that may be needed for older women and older adults from racial and ethnic minority groups.

10
Further Reading

Areán, P. A. (Ed.). (2016). *Treatment of late-life depression, anxiety, trauma, and substance abuse.* American Psychological Association.
This book covers specific treatments for mental health conditions among older adults, including three chapters devoted to substance use (brief interventions, SBIRT, and relapse prevention). Other chapters provide useful information on treatments for late life depression and anxiety.

Han, B. H., & Moore, A. A. (2018). Prevention and screening of unhealthy substance use by older adults. *Clinics in Geriatric Medicine, 34*(1), 117–129. https://doi.org/10.1016/j.cger.2017.08.005
This article is particularly useful in understanding why the current DSM-5 criteria for alcohol use disorders (AUDs) may be problematic for older adults. It also offers practical strategies for alcohol screening among older adults, and recommends specific screening instruments.

Kuerbis, A., Moore, A., Sacco, P., & Zanjani, F. (Eds.). (2016). *Alcohol and aging: Clinical and public health perspectives.* Springer.
An in-depth book covering many specific aspects of substance use and older adults, including topics such as social and family contexts around drinking, elder abuse and drinking, alcohol and health conditions, and alcohol and cognition.

Substance Abuse and Mental Health Services Administration. (2020). *Treating substance use disorder in older adults. Treatment Improvement Protocol (TIP)* (Series No. 26, SAMHSA Publication No. PEP20-02-01-011).
This publication provides detailed information on assessment and treatment options for older adults who present with a range of severity of unhealthy alcohol use. Specific clinical examples are provided for many treatment approaches.

References

Aalto, M., Alho, H., Halme, J. T., & Seppä, K. (2011). The alcohol use disorders identification test (AUDIT) and its derivatives in screening for heavy drinking among the elderly. *Journal of Geriatric Psychiatry, 26*(9), 881–885. https://doi.org/10.1002/gps.2498

Administration for Community Living. (2021). *2020 Profile of older Americans.* https://acl.gov/aging-and-disability-in-america/data-and-research/profile-older-americans

American Psychiatric Association. (2013). *Diagnostic and statistical manual of mental disorders* (5th ed.). https://doi.org/10.1176/appi.books.9780890425596

Amirkhan, J., & Auyeung, B. (2007). Coping with stress across the lifespan: Absolute vs. relative changes in strategy. *Journal of Applied Developmental Psychology, 28*(4), 298–317. https://doi.org/10.1016/j.appdev.2007.04.002

Andrabi, N., Khoddam, R., & Leventhal, A. M. (2017). Socioeconomic disparities in adolescent substance use: Role of enjoyable alternative substance-free activities. *Social Science & Medicine, 176,* 175–182. https://doi.org/10.1016/j.socscimed.2016.12.032

Assari, S., & Moghani Lankarani, M. (2016). Education and alcohol consumption among older Americans: Black-white differences. *Frontiers in Public Health, 4,* 67. https://doi.org/10.3389/fpubh.2016.00067

Assari, S., Smith, J., Mistry, R., Farokhnia, M., & Bazargan, M. (2019). Substance use among economically disadvantaged African American older adults: Objective and subjective socioeconomic status. *International Journal of Environmental Research and Public Health, 16*(10), 1826. https://doi.org/10.3390/ijerph16101826

Australian Bureau of Statistics National Health Survey. (2009). *Summary of results, 2007-2008.* https://www.abs.gov.au/ausstats/abs@.nsf/mf/4364.0/

Bahorik, A. L., Leibowitz, A., Sterling, S. A., Travis, A., Weisner, C., & Satre, D. D. (2016). The role of hazardous drinking in predicting depression and anxiety symptom improvement among psychiatry patients: A longitudinal study. *Journal of Affective Disorders, 206,* 169–173. https://doi.org/10.1016/j.jad.2016.07.039

Barry, K. L., & Blow, F. C. (2016). Drinking over the lifespan: Focus on older adults. *Alcohol Research: Current Reviews, 38*(1), 115–120.

Bernal, G., Jiménez-Chafey, M. I., & Domenech Rodríguez, M. M. (2009). Cultural adaptation of treatments: A resource for considering culture in evidence-based practice. *Professional Psychology: Research and Practice, 40*(4), 361–368. https://doi.org/10.1037/a0016401

Birditt, K. S., Polenick, C. A., Luong, G., Charles, S. T., & Fingerman, K. L. (2020). Daily interpersonal tensions and well-being among older adults: The role of emotion regulations strategies. *Psychology and Aging, 35*(4), 578–590. https://doi.org/10.1037/pag0000416

Blow, F. C., Brower, K. J., Schulenberg, J. E., Demo-Dananberg, L. M., Young, J. P., & Beresford, T. P. (1991). The Michigan Alcoholism Screening Test-Geriatric Version (MAST-G): A new elderly specific screening instrument. *Alcoholism: Clinical and Experimental Research, 16*(2), 372.

Boersma, P., Black, L. I., & Ward, B. W. (2020). Prevalence of multiple chronic conditions among US Adults, 2018. *Preventing Chronic Disease, 17,* 200130. https://doi.org/10.5888/pcd17.200130

Brennan, P.L., Holland, J.M., Schutte, K.K., & Moos, R.H. (2012). Drinking trajectories in later life: A 20-year predictive study. *Aging and Mental Health, 16*(3), 305-316. https://doi.org/10.1080/13607863.2011.628975

Breslow, R.A., Castle, I.-J.P., Chen, C.M., & Graubard, B.I. (2017). Trends in alcohol consumption among older Americans: National health interview surveys, 1997-2014. *Alcohol: Clinical and Experimental Research, 41*(5), 976-986. https://doi.org/10.1111/acer.13365

Breslow, R.A., Dong, C., & White, A. (2015). Prevalence of alcohol-interactive prescription medication use among current drinkers: United States, 1999-2010. *Alcoholism: Clinical and Experimental Research, 39*(2), 371-379. https://doi.org/10.1111/acer.12633

Burrow-Sánchez, J.J., & Nielsen, M. (2020). Screening, brief intervention, and referral to treatment for racial and ethnic minority populations: State of the science and implications for adaptation. In M.D. Cimini & J.L. Martin (Eds.), *Screening, brief intervention, and referral to treatment for substance use: A practitioner's guide* (pp. 161-177). American Psychological Association. https://doi.org/10.1037/0000199-010

Bush, K., Kivlahan, D.R., McDonell, M.B., Fihn, S.D., Bradley, K.A., & Ambulatory Care Quality Improvement Project (ACQUIP). (1998). The AUDIT alcohol consumption questions (AUDIT-C): An effective brief screening test for problem drinking. *Archives of Internal Medicine, 158*(16), 1789-1795. https://doi.org/10.1001/archinte.158.16.1789

Camicia, M., Chamberlain, B., Finnie, R.R., Nalle, M., Lindeke, L.L., Lorenz, L., Hain, D., Haney, K.D., Campbell-Heider, N., Pecenka-Johnson, K., Jones, T., Parker-Guyton, N., Brydges, G., Briggs, W.T., Cisco, M.C., Haney, C., & McMenamin, P. (2013). The value of nursing care coordination: A white paper of the American Nurses Association. *Nursing Outlook, 61,* 491-501. https://doi.org/10.1016/j.outlook.2013.10.006

Caputo, F., Vignoli, T., Leggio, L., Addolorato, G., Zoli, G., & Bernardi, M. (2012). Alcohol use disorders in the elderly: A brief overview from epidemiology to treatment options. *Experimental Gerontology, 47*(6), 411-416. https://doi.org/10.1016/j.exger.2012.03.019

Catley, D., Harris, K.J., Mayo, M.S., Hall, S., Okuyemi, K.S., Boardman, T., & Ahluwalia, J.S. (2006). Adherence to principles of motivational interviewing and client within-session behavior. *Behavioural and Cognitive Psychotherapy, 34*(1), 43-56. https://doi.org/10.1017/S1352465805002432

Center for Substance Abuse Treatment. (2005). *Substance abuse relapse prevention for older adults: A group treatment approach* (DHHS Publication No. (SMA) 05-4053). Substance Abuse and Mental Health Services Administration.

Chan, K.K., Neighbors, C., Gilson, M., Larimer, M.E., & Marlatt, G.A. (2007). Epidemiological trends in drinking by age and gender: Providing normative feedback to adults. *Addictive Behaviors, 32*(5), 967-976. https://doi.org/10.1016/j.addbeh.2006.07.003

Chen, J.A., Glass, J.E., Bensley, K.M.K., Goldberg, S.B., Lehavot, K., & Williams, E.C. (2020). Racial/ethnic and gender differences in receipt of brief intervention among patients with unhealthy alcohol use in the U.S. Veterans Health Administration. *Journal of Substance Abuse Treatment, 119,* 108078. https://doi.org/10.1016/j.jsat.2020.108078

Choi, N.G., & DiNitto, D.M. (2019). Older marijuana users in substance abuse treatment: Treatment settings for marijuana-only versus polysubstance use admissions. *Journal of Substance Abuse Treatment, 105,* 28-36. https://doi.org/10.1016/j.jsat.2019.07.016

Choi, N.G., DiNitto, D.M., & Marti, C.N. (2014). Treatment use, perceived need, and barriers to seeking treatment for substance abuse and mental health problems among older adults compared to younger adults. *Drug and Alcohol Dependence, 145*, 113–120. https://doi.org/10.1016/j.drugalcdep.2014.10.004

Choi, N.G., DiNitto, D.M., & Marti, C.N. (2016). Older-adult marijuana users and ex-users: Comparisons of sociodemographic characteristics and mental and substance use disorders. *Drug and Alcohol Dependence, 165*, 94–102. https://doi.org/10.1016/j.drugalcdep.2016.05.023

Choi, N.G., DiNitto, D.M., Sagna, A.O., & Marti, C.N. (2018). Postmortem blood alcohol content among late-middle aged and older suicide decedents: Associations with suicide precipitating/risk factors, means, and other drug toxicology. *Drug and Alcohol Dependence, 187*, 311–318. https://doi.org/10.1016/j.drugalcdep.2018.02.034

Cook, J.M., McCarthy, E., & Thorp, S.R. (2017). Older adults with PTSD: Brief state of research and evidence-based psychotherapy case illustration. *American Journal of Geriatric Psychiatry, 5*, 522–530. https://doi.org/10.1016/j.jagp.2016.12.016

Coon, D.W., & Thompson, L.W. (2003). The relationship between homework compliance and treatment outcomes among older adult outpatients with mild-to-moderate depression. *American Journal of Geriatric Psychiatry, 11*(1), 53–61. https://doi.org/10.1097/00019442-200301000-00008

Crummy, E.A., O'Neal, T.J., Baskin, B.M., & Ferguson, S.M. (2020). One is not enough: Understanding and modeling polysubstance use. *Frontiers in Neuroscience, 14*. https://doi.org/10.3389/fnins.2020.00569

Cummings, S.M., Cooper, R.L., & McClure Cassie, K. (2009). Motivational interviewing to affect behavioral change in older adults. *Research on Social Work Practice, 19*(2), 195–204. https://doi.org/10.1177/1049731508320216

Dar, K. (2006). Alcohol use disorders in elderly people: Fact or fiction? *Advances in Psychiatric Treatment, 12*(3), 173–181. https://doi.org/10.1192/apt.12.3.173

DeMarce, J.M., Gnys, M., Raffa, S.D., & Karlin, B.E. (2014). *Cognitive behavioral therapy for substance use disorders among veterans: Therapist manual.* US Department of Veterans Affairs.

Dreher-Weber, M., Laireiter, A.-R., Kühberger, A., Kunz, I., Yegles, M., Binz, T., Rumpf, H.-J., Hoffman, R., Praxenthaler, V., Lang, S., & Wurst, F.M. (2017). Screening for hazardous drinking in nursing home residents: Evaluating the validity of the current cut-offs of the Alcohol Use Disorder Identification Test – Consumption questions by using ethyl glucuronide in hair. *Alcoholism: Clinical and Experimental Research, 41*(9), 1593–1601. https://doi.org/10.1111/acer.13449

Dupree, L.W., Broskowski, H., & Schonfeld, L. (1984). The Gerontology Alcohol Project: A behavioral treatment program for elderly alcohol abusers. *The Gerontologist, 24*(5), 510–516. https://doi.org/10.1093/geront/24.5.510

Emiliussen, J., Andersen, K., & Nielsen, A.S. (2017). Why do some older adults start drinking excessively late in life? Results from an Interpretative Phenomenological Study. *Scandinavian Journal of Caring Sciences, 31*, 974–983. https://doi.org/10.1111/scs.12421

Epstein, E.E., Fischer-Elber, K., Al-Otaiba, Z. (2007). Women, aging, and alcohol use disorders. *Journal of Women & Aging, 19*(1-2), 31–48. https://doi.org/10.1300/J074v19n01_03

Epstein, E.E., McCrady, B.S., Hallgren, K.A., Cook, S., Jensen, N.K., & Hildebrandt, T. (2018). A randomized trial of female-specific cognitive behavior therapy for alcohol dependent women. *Psychology of Addictive Behaviors, 32*(1), 1–15. https://doi.org/10.1037/adb0000330

Epstein, E. E., McCrady, B. S., Hallgren, K. A., Gaba, A., Cook, S., Jensen, N., Hildebrandt, T., Holzhauer, C. G., & Litt, M. D. (2018). Individual versus group female-specific cognitive behavior therapy for alcohol use disorder. *Journal of Substance Abuse Treatment, 88,* 27–43. https://doi.org/10.1016/j.jsat.2018.02.003

Ettner, S. L., Xu, H., Kenrik Duru, O., Ang, A., Tseng, C.-H., Tallen, L., Barnes, A., Mirkin, M., Ransohoff, K., & Moore, A. A. (2014). The effect of an educational intervention on alcohol consumption, at-risk drinking, and health care utilization in older adults: The Project SHARE study. *Journal of Studies on Alcohol and Drugs, 75*(3), 447–457. https://doi.org/10.15288/jsad.2014.75.447

Ferreira, M. P., & Weems, M. K. S. (2008). Alcohol consumption by aging adults in the United States: Health benefits and detriments. *Journal of the American Dietetic Association, 108*(10), 1668–1676. https://doi.org/10.1016/j.jada.2008.07.011

Fleming, M. F., Manwell, L. B., Barry, K. L., Adams, W., & Stauffacher, E. A. (1999). Brief physician advice for alcohol problems in older adults: A randomized community-based trial. *Journal of Family Practice, 48,* 378–386.

French, D. J., Sargent-Cox, K. A., Kim, S., & Anstey, K. J. (2014). Gender differences in alcohol consumption among middle-aged and older adults in Australia, the United States and Korea. *Australian and New Zealand Journal of Public Health, 38*(4), 332–339. https://doi.org/10.1111/1753-6405.12227

Frost, H., Campbell, P., Maxwell, M., O'Carroll, R. E., Dombrowski, S. U., Williams, B., Cheyne, H., Coles, E., & Pollock, A. (2018). Effectiveness of Motivational Interviewing on adult behaviour change in health and social care settings: A systematic review of reviews. *PLOS One, 13*(10), e0204890. https://doi.org/10.1371/journal.pone.0204890

Gell, L., Meier, P. S., & Goyder, E. (2015). Alcohol consumption among the over 50s: International comparisons. *Alcohol and Alcoholism, 50*(1), 1–10. https://doi.org/10.1093/alcalc/agu082

Goldhammer, H., Krinsky, L., & Keuroghlian, A. S. (2019). Meeting the behavioral health needs of LGBT older adults. *Journal of the American Geriatric Society, 67*(8), 1565–1570. https://doi.org/10.1111/jgs.15974

Gómez, A., Conde, A., Santana, J. M., Jorrín, A., Serrano, I. M., & Medina, R. (2006). The diagnostic usefulness of AUDIT and AUDIT-C for detecting hazardous drinkers in the elderly. *Aging and Mental Health, 10*(5), 558–561. https://doi.org/10.1080/13607860600637729

Goodman, R. (2017). Contemporary trauma theory and trauma-informed care in substance use disorders: A conceptual model for integrating coping and resilience. *Advances in Social Work, 18*(1), 186–201. https://doi.org/10.18060/21312

Gordon, A. J., Conigliaro, J., Maisto, S. A., McNeil, M., Kraemer, K. L., & Kelley, M. E. (2003). Comparison of consumption effects of brief interventions for hazardous drinking elderly. *Substance Use & Misuse, 8,* 1017–1035. https://doi.org/10.1081/JA-120017649

Grant, B. F., Chou, S. P., Saha, T. D., Pickering, R. P., Kerridge, B. T., Ruan, W. J., Huang, B., Jung, J., Zhang, H., Fan, A., & Hasin, D. (2017). Prevalence of 12-month alcohol use, high-risk drinking, and DSM-IV alcohol use disorder in the United States, 2001–2002 to 2012–2013: Results from the National Epidemiologic Survey on Alcohol and Related Conditions. *JAMA Psychiatry, 74*(9), 911–923. https://doi.org/10.1001/jamapsychiatry.2017.2161

Grant, B.F., Hasin, D.S., Chou, S.P., Stinson, F.S., & Dawson, D.A. (2004). Nicotine dependence and psychiatric disorders in the United States: Results from the National Epidemiologic Survey on Alcohol and Related Conditions. *Archives of General Psychiatry, 61*(11), 1107–1115. https://doi.org/10.1001/archpsyc.61.11.1107

Green, H.D. (2018). A community-based evaluation of screening, brief intervention, and referral to treatment (SBIRT) for the Black community. *Qualitative Health Research, 28*(3), 418–432. https://doi.org/10.1177/1049732317746962

Han, B.H. (2019). Aging, multimorbidity, and substance use disorders: The growing case for integrating the principles of geriatric care and harm reduction. *International Journal of Drug Policy, 58,* 135–136. https://doi.org/10.1016/j.drugpo.2018.06.005

Han, B.H., Miyoshi, M., & Palamar, J.J. (2020). Substance use among middle-aged and older lesbian, gay, and bisexual adults in the United States, 2015–2017. *Journal of General Internal Medicine, 35,* 3740–3741. https://doi.org/10.1007/s11606-020-05635-2

Han, B.H., & Moore, A.A. (2018). Prevention and screening of unhealthy substance use by older adults. *Clinics in Geriatric Medicine, 34*(1), 117–129. https://doi.org/10.1016/j.cger.2017.08.005

Han, B.H., Moore, A.A., Sherman, S., Keyes, K.M., & Palamar, J.J. (2017). Demographic trends of binge alcohol use and alcohol use disorders among older adults in the United States, 2005–2014. *Drug and Alcohol Dependence, 170,* 198–207. https://doi.org/10.1016/j.drugalcdep.2016.11.003

Han, B.H., & Palamar, J.J. (2020). Trends in cannabis use among older adults in the United States, 2015–2018. *JAMA Internal Medicine, 180*(4), 609–611. https://doi.org/10.1001/jamainternmed.2019.7517

Hanson, M., & Gutheil, I.A. (2004). Motivational strategies with alcohol-involved older adults: Implications for social work practice. *Social Work, 49*(3), 364–372. https://doi.org/10.1093/sw/49.3.364

Harada, C.N., Natelson Love, M.C., & Triebel, K.L. (2013). Normal cognitive aging. *Clinics in Geriatric Medicine, 29*(4), P737–P752. https://doi.org/10.1016/j.cger.2013.07.002

Henley, S.J., Asman, K., Momin, B., Gallaway, M.S., Culp, M.B., Ragan, K.R., Richards, T.B., & Babb, S. (2019). Smoking cessation behaviors among older U.S. adults. *Preventive Medicine Reports, 16,* 100978. https://doi.org/10.1016/j.pmedr.2019.100978

Higgins, S.T., Heil, S.H., & Peck, K.R. (2021). Substance use disorders. In D.H. Barlow (Ed.), *Clinical handbook of psychological disorders* (6th ed., pp. 612–637). Guilford Press.

Highland, K.B., Herschel, L.C., Klanecky, A., & McChargue, D.E. (2013). Biopsychosocial pathways to alcohol-related problems. *American Journal on Addictions, 22*(4), 366–372. https://doi.org/10.1111/j.1521-0391.2013.12012.x

Holland, J.M., Rozalski, V., Beckman, L., Rakhkovskaya, L.M., Klingspon, K.L., Donohue, B., Williams, C., Thompson, L.W., & Gallagher-Thompson, D. (2016). Treatment preferences of older adults with substance use problems. *Clinical Gerontologist, 39*(1), 15–24. https://doi.org/10.1080/07317115.2015.1101633

Horvath, A.T., & Yeterian, J.D. (2012). SMART Recovery: Self-empowering, science-based addiction recovery support. *Journal of Groups in Addiction and Recovery, 7,* 102–117. https://doi.org/10.1080/1556035X.2012.705651

Immonen, S., Valvanne, J., & Pitkälä, K.H. (2010). Older adults' own reasoning for their alcohol consumption. *International Journal of Geriatric Psychiatry, 26*(11), 1169–1176. https://doi.org/10.1002/gps.2657

Isenberg-Grzeda, E., Kutner, H. E., & Nicolson, S. E. (2012). Wernicke-Korsakoff-Syndrome: Under-recognized and under-treated. *Psychosomatics, 53*(6), 507–516. https://doi.org/10.1016/j.psym.2012.04.008

Jamal, A., King, B. A., Neff, L. J., Whitmill, J., Babb, S. D., & Graffunder, C. M. (2016). *Current cigarette smoking among adults – United States,* 2005–2015. *Morbidity and Mortality Weekly Report, 65*(44), 1205–1211. https://doi.org/10.15585/mmwr.mm6544a2

Johnson, S. F., Barrera, K., & Yochim, B. P. (2018). Cognition and aging. In B. P. Yochim & E. L. Woodhead (Eds.), *Psychology of aging: A biopsychosocial perspective* (pp. 157–175). Springer.

Källmén, H., Wennberg, P., Ramstedt, M., & Hallgren, M. (2014). Psychometric properties of the AUDIT: A survey from a random sample of elderly Swedish adults. *BMC Public Health, 14,* 672. https://doi.org/10.1186/1471-2458-14-672

Kaskutas, L. A., Subbaraman, M., Witbrodt, J., & Zemore, S. (2009). Effectiveness of making alcoholics anonymous easier: A group format 12-step facilitation approach. *Journal of Substance Abuse Treatment, 37*(3), 228–239. https://doi.org/10.1016/j.jsat.2009.01.004

Kelly, J. F., Saitz, R., & Wakeman, S. (2016). Language, substance use disorders, and policy: The need to reach consensus on an "Addiction-ary." *Alcoholism Treatment, 34*(1), 116–123. https://doi.org/10.1080/07347324.2016.1113103

Kelly, J. F., Humphreys, K., & Ferri, M. (2020). Alcoholic Anonymous and other 12-step programs for alcohol use disorder. *Cochrane Database of Systematic Reviews, 3,* CD012880. https://doi.org/10.1002/14651858.CD012880.pub2

Kelly, J. F., & McCrady, B. S. (2008). Twelve-step facilitation in non-specialty settings. In L. Kaskutas & M. Galanter (Eds.). *Recent developments in alcoholism: Research on Alcoholics Anonymous and spirituality in addiction recovery* (Vol. 18, pp. 321–346). Springer. https://doi.org/10.1007/978-0-387-77725-2_18

Kerr, W. C., & Stockwell, T. (2012). Understanding standard drinks and drinking guidelines. *Drug and Alcohol Review, 31*(2), 200–205. https://doi.org/10.1111/j.1465-3362.2011.00374.x

Kist, N., Sandjojo, J., Kok, R. M., & van den Berg, J. F. (2014). Cognitive functioning in older adults with early, late, and very late onset alcohol dependence. *International Psychogeriatrics, 26*(11), 1863–1869. https://doi.org/10.1017/S1041610214000878

Knightly, R., Tadros, G., Sharma, J., Duffield, P., Carnall, E., Fisher, J., & Salman, S. (2016). Alcohol screening for older adults in an acute general hospital: FAST v. MAST-G assessments. *BJPsych Bulletin, 40*(2), 72–76. https://doi.org/10.1192/pb.bp.114.049734

Kroenke, K., Spitzer, R. L., & Williams, J. B. W. (2001). The PHQ-9: Validity of a brief depression severity measure. *Journal of General Internal Medicine, 16*(9), 606–613. https://doi.org/10.1046/j.1525-1497.2001.016009606.x

Kuerbis, A. (2020). Substance use among older adults: Prevalence, etiology, assessment, and intervention. *Gerontology, 66,* 249–258. https://doi.org/10.1159/000504363

Kuerbis, A. N., Hagman, B. T., & Sacco, P. (2013). Functioning of alcohol use disorders criteria among middle-aged and older adults: Implications for DSM-5. *Substance Use & Misuse, 48*(4), 309–322. https://doi.org/10.3109/10826084.2012.762527

Kuerbis, A. N., & Sacco, P. (2012). The impact of retirement on the drinking patterns of older adults: A review. *Addictive Behaviors, 37*(5), 587–595. https://doi.org/10.1016/j.addbeh.2012.01.022

Kuerbis, A.N., Sacco, P., Blazer, D.G., & Moore, A.A. (2014). Substance abuse among older adults. *Clinics in Geriatric Medicine, 30*(3), 629–654. https://doi.org/10.1016/j.cger.2014.04.008

Lee, C.S., Colby, S.M., Rohsenow, D.J., Martin, R., Rosales, R., McCallum, T.T., Falcon, L., Almeida, J., & Cortés, D.E. (2019). A randomized controlled trial of motivational interviewing tailored for heavy drinking latinxs. *Journal of Consulting and Clinical Psychology, 87*(9), 815–830. https://doi.org/10.1037/ccp0000428

Lee, M.R., & Sher, K.J. (2018). "Maturing out" of binge and problem drinking. *Alcohol Research: Current Reviews, 39*(1), 31–42.

Leggat, G., Livingston, M., Kuntsche, S., & Callinan, S. (2021). Changes in alcohol consumption during pregnancy and over the transition towards parenthood. *Drug and Alcohol Dependence, 225*, Article 108745. https://doi.org/10.1016/j.drugalcdep.2021.108745

Lehman, B.J., David, D.M., & Gruber, J.A. (2017). Rethinking the biopsychosocial model of health: Understanding health as a dynamic system. *Social and Personality Psychology Compass, 11*(8), https://doi.org/10.1111/spc3.12328

Magill, M., Apodaca, T.R., Borsari, B., Gaume, J., Hoadley, A., Gordon, R.E. F., Tonigan, J.S., & Moyers, T. (2018). A meta-analysis of motivational interviewing process: Technical, relational, and conditional process models of change. *Journal of Consulting and Clinical Psychology, 86*(2), 140–157. https://doi.org/10.1037/ccp0000250

Magill, M., & Hallgren, K.A. (2019). Mechanisms of behavior change in motivational interviewing: Do we understand how MI works? *Current Opinion in Psychology, 30*, 1–5. https://doi.org/10.1016/j.copsyc.2018.12.010

Malczyk, E., Dzięgielewska-Gęsiak, S., Fatyga, E., Ziółko, E., Kokot, T. & Muc-Wierzgoń, M. (2016). Body composition in healthy older persons: Role of the ratio of extracellular/total body water. *Journal of Biological Regulators and Homeostatic Agents, 30*(3), 447–452.

Manuel, J.K., Satre, D.D., Tsoh, J., Moreno-John, G., Ramos, J.S., McCance-Katz, E.F., & Satterfield, J.M. (2015). Adapting Screening, Brief Intervention, and Referral to Treatment (SBIRT) for alcohol and drugs to culturally diverse clinical populations. *Journal of Addiction Medicine, 9*(5), 343–351. https://doi.org/10.1097/ADM.0000000000000150

McCrady, B., Wilson, A., Muñoz, R., Fink, B., Fokas, K., & Borders, A. (2016). Alcohol-focused behavioral couple therapy. *Family Process, 55*(3), 443–459. https://doi.org/10.1111/famp.12231

McCrady, D.S., & Epstein, E.E. (2021). Alcohol use disorders. In D.H. Barlow (Ed.), *Clinical handbook of psychological disorders* (6th ed., pp. 555–611). Guilford Press.

Miller, W.R., & Rollnick, S. (2013). *Motivational interviewing: Helping people change* (3rd ed.). Guilford.

Moore, A.A., Blow, F.C., Hoffing, M., Welgreen, S., Davis, J.W., Lin, J.C., Ramirez, K.D., Liao, D.H., Tang, L., Gould, R., Gill, M., Chen, O., & Barry, K.L. (2011). Primary care-based intervention to reduce at-risk drinking in older adults: A randomized controlled trial. *Addiction, 106*(1), 111–120. https://doi.org/10.1111/j.1360-0443.2010.03229.x

Moos, R.H. (2007). Theory-based processes that promote the remission of substance use disorders. *Clinical Psychology Review, 27*(5), 537–551. https://doi.org/10.1016/j.cpr.2006.12.006

Moos, R. H., Schutte, K. K., Brennan, P. L., & Moos, B. S. (2010). Late-life and life history predictors of older adults of high-risk alcohol consumption and drinking problems. *Drug and Alcohol Dependence, 108*(1-2), 13-20. https://doi.org/10.1016/j.drugalcdep.2009.11.005

National Institute on Alcohol Abuse and Alcoholism. (2014). *Mixing alcohol with medications.* https://www.niaaa.nih.gov/publications/brochures-and-fact-sheets/harmful-interactions-mixing-alcohol-with-medicines

National Institute on Alcohol Abuse and Alcoholism. (2018). Drinking patterns and their definitions. *Alcohol Research: Current Reviews, 39*(1). https://arcr.niaaa.nih.gov/binge-drinking-predictors-patterns-and-consequences/drinking-patterns-and-their-definitions

National Institute on Alcohol Abuse and Alcoholism. (2021). *Understanding binge drinking.* https://www.niaaa.nih.gov/publications/brochures-and-fact-sheets/binge-drinking

Orgeta, V., Brede, J., & Livingston, G. (2017). Behavioural activation for depression in older people: Systematic review and meta-analysis. *British Journal of Psychiatry, 211*(5), 274-279. https://doi.org/10.1192/bjp.bp.117.205021

Ornelas, I. J., Allen, C., Vaughan, C., Williams, E. C., & Negi, N. (2015). Vida PURA: A cultural adaptation of screening and brief intervention to reduce unhealthy drinking among Latino day laborers. *Substance Abuse, 36*(3), 264-271. https://doi.org/10.1080/08897077.2014.955900

Oslin, D., Liberto, J. G., O'Brien, J., Krois, S., & Norbeck, J. (1997). Naltrexone as an adjunctive treatment for older patients with alcohol dependence. *American Journal of Geriatric Psychiatry, 5*(4), 324-332. https://doi.org/10.1097/00019442-199700540-00007

Oslin, D. W., Pettinati, H., & Volpicelli, J. R. (2002). Alcoholism treatment adherence: Older age predicts better adherence and drinking outcomes. *American Journal of Geriatric Psychiatry, 10*(6), 740-747. https://doi.org/10.1097/00019442-200211000-00013

Oslin, D. W., Slaymaker, V. J., Blow, F. C., Owen, P. L., & Colleran, C. (2005). Treatment outcomes for alcohol dependence among middle-aged and older adults. *Addictive Behaviors, 30*(7), 1431-1436. https://doi.org/10.1016/j.addbeh.2005.01.007

Parish, W. J., Mark, T. L., Weber, E. M., & Steinberg, D. G. (2022). Substance use disorders among Medicare beneficiaries: Prevalence, mental and physical comorbidities, and treatment barriers. *American Journal of Preventive Medicine, 63*(2), P225-P232. https://doi.org/10.1016/j.amepre.2022.01.021

Park, S.-Y., Anastas, J., Shibusawa, T., & Nguyen, D. (2014). The impact of acculturation and acculturative stress on alcohol use across Asian immigrant subgroups. *Substance Use and Misuse, 8*, 922-931. https://doi.org/10.3109/10826084.2013.855232

Parlesak, A., Billinger, M. H., Bode, C., & Bode, J. C. (2002). Gastric alcohol dehydrogenase activity in man: Influence of gender, age, alcohol consumption and smoking in a Caucasian population. *Alcohol and Alcoholism, 37*(4), 388-393. https://doi.org/10.1093/alcalc/37.4.388

Peele, S. (2016). People control their addictions: No matter how much the "chronic" brain disease model of addiction indicates otherwise, we know that people can quit addictions – with special reference to harm reduction and mindfulness. *Addictive Behaviors Reports, 4*, 97-101. https://doi.org/10.1016/j.abrep.2016.05.003

Peltier, M. R., Verplaetse, T. L., Mineur, Y. S., Petrakis, I. L., Cosgrove, K. P., Picciotti, M. R., & McKee, S. A. (2019). Sex differences in stress-related alcohol use. *Neurobiology of Stress, 10*, 100149. https://doi.org/10.1016/j.ynstr.2019.100149

Rao, R., Schofield, P., & Ashworth, M. (2015). Alcohol use, socioeconomic deprivation and ethnicity in older people. *BMJ Open, 5*(8). https://doi.org/10.1136/bmjopen-2014-007525

Rice, C., Longabaugh, R., Beattie, M., & Noel, N. (1993). Age groups differences in response to treatment for problematic alcohol use. *Addiction, 88*(10), 1369–1375. https://doi.org/10.1111/j.1360-0443.1993.tb02023.x

Rider, K. L., Thompson, L. W., & Gallagher-Thompson, D. (2016). California Older Persons Pleasant Events Scale: A tool to help older adults increase positive experiences. *Clinical Gerontologist, 39*(1), 64–83. https://doi.org/10.1080/07317115.2015.1101635

Roozen, H. G., De Waart, R., & Van Der Kroft, P. (2010). Community reinforcement and family training: An effective option to engage treatment-resistant substance-abusing individuals in treatment. *Addiction, 105*(10), 1729–1738. https://doi.org/10.1111/j.1360-0443.2010.03016.x

Rubak, S., Sandbæk, A., Lauritzen, T., & Christensen, B. (2005). Motivational interviewing: A systematic review and meta-analysis. *Journal of General Practice, 55*(513), 305–312.

Rubin, A., Parrish, D. E., & Miyawaki, C. E. (2019). Benchmarks for evaluating life review and reminiscence therapy in alleviating depression among older adults. *Social Work, 64*(1), 61–72. https://doi.org/10.1093/sw/swy054

Sacco, P., Bucholz, K. K., & Harrington, D. (2014). Gender differences in stressful life events, social support, perceived stress, and alcohol use among older adults: Results from a national survey. *Substance Use & Misuse, 49*(4), 456–465. https://doi.org/10.3109/10826084.2013.846379

Sacco, P., Burruss, K., Smith, C. A., Kuerbis, A., Harrington, D., Moore, A. A., & Resnick, B. (2015). Drinking behavior among older adults at a continuing care retirement community: Affective and motivational influences. *Aging & Mental Health, 19*(3), 279–289. https://doi.org/10.1080/13607863.2014.933307

Saitz, R. (2005). Unhealthy alcohol use. *New England Journal of Medicine, 352*, 596–607. https://doi.org/10.1056/NEJMcp042262

Salthouse, T. A. (2010). Selective review of cognitive aging. *Journal of the International Neuropsychological Society, 16*(5), 754–760. https://doi.org/10.1017/S135561771000706

Satre, D. D., Chi, F. W., Mertens, J. R., & Weisner, C. M. (2012). Effects of age and life transitions on alcohol and drug treatment outcome over nine years. *Journal of Studies on Alcohol and Drugs, 73*(3), 459–468. https://doi.org/10.15288/jsad.2012.73.459

Satre, D. D., Gordon, N. P., & Weisner, C. (2007). Alcohol consumption, medical conditions and health behavior among older adults. *American Journal of Health Behavior, 31*(3), 238–248. https://doi.org/10.5993/AJHB.31.3.2

Satre, D. D., Manuel, J. K., Larios, S., Steiger, S., & Satterfield, J. (2015). Clinical case conference: Cultural adaptation of screening, brief intervention and referral to treatment (SBIRT) using Motivational Interviewing. *Journal of Addiction Medicine, 9*(5), 352–357. https://doi.org/10.1097/ADM.0000000000000149

Satre, D. D., Mertens, J. R., Areán, P. A., & Weisner, C. (2003). Contrasting outcomes of older versus middle-aged and younger adult chemical dependency patients in a managed care program. *Journal of Studies on Alcohol and Drugs, 64*(4), 520–530. https://doi.org/10.15288/jsa.2003.64.520

Satre, D.D., Mertens, J.R., Areán, P.A., & Weisner, C. (2004). Five-year alcohol and drug treatment outcomes of older adults versus middle-aged and younger adults in a managed care program. *Addiction, 99*(10), 1286–1297. https://doi.org/10.1111/j.1360-0443.2004.00831.x

Satre, D.D., Mertens, J.R., & Weisner, C. (2004). Gender differences in treatment outcomes for alcohol dependence among older adults. *Journal of Studies on Alcohol and Drugs, 65*(5), 638–642. https://doi.org/10.15288/jsa.2004.65.638

Saunders, J.B., Aasland, O.G., Babor, T.F., De La Fuente, J.R., & Grant, M. (1993). Development of the Alcohol Use Disorders Identification Test (AUDIT): WHO Collaborative Project on Early Detection of Persons with Harmful Alcohol Consumption – II. *Addiction, 88*(6), 791–804. https://doi.org/10.1111/j.1360-0443.1993.tb02093.x

Schaie, K.W. (1994). The course of adult intellectual development. *American Psychologist, 49*(4), 304–313. https://doi.org/10.1037/0003-066X.49.4.304

Schonfeld, L. (2020). Screening, brief intervention, and referral to treatment for older adults: Lessons learned from the Florida BRITE Project. In M.D. Cimini & J.L. Martin (Eds.), *Screening, brief intervention, and referral to treatment for substance use: A practitioner's guide* (pp. 179–197). American Psychological Association. https://doi.org/10.1037/0000199-011

Schonfeld, L., Dupree, L.W., Dickson-Fuhrmann, E., McKean Royer, C., McDermott, C.H., Rosansky, J.S., Taylor, S., & Jarvik, L.F. (2000). Cognitive-behavioral treatment for older veterans with substance abuse problems. *Journal of Geriatric Psychiatry and Neurology, 13*(3), 124–129. https://doi.org/10.1177/089198870001300305

Schonfeld, L., King-Kallimanis, B.L., Duchene, D.M., Etheridge, R.L., Herrera, J.R., Barry, K.L., & Lynn, N. (2010). Screening and brief intervention for substance misuse among older adults: The Florida BRITE project. *American Journal of Public Health, 100*(1), 108–114. https://doi.org/10.2105/AJPH.2008.149534

Self, K.J., Borsari, B., Ladd, B.O., Nicolas, G., Gibson, C.J., Jackson, K., & Manuel, J.K. (2022). Cultural adaptations of motivational interviewing: A systematic review. *Psychological Services.* Advance online publication. http://doi.org/10.1037/ser0000619

Shaw, B.A., Ahagi, N., & Krause, N. (2011). Are changes in financial strain associated with changes in alcohol use and smoking among older adults? *Journal of Studies on Alcohol and Drugs, 72*(6), 917–925. https://doi.org/10.15288/jsad.2011.72.917

Skewes, M.C., & Gonzalez, V.M. (2013). The biopsychosocial model of addiction. In P.M. Miller (Ed.), *Principles of addition: Comprehensive addiction behaviors and disorders* (Vol. 1, pp. 61–70). Elsevier. https://doi.org/10.1016/C2011-0-07778-5

Slade, T., Chapman, C., Swift, W., Keyes, K., Tonks, Z., & Teesson, M. (2016). Birth cohort trends in the global epidemiology of alcohol use and alcohol-related harms in men and women: Systematic review and metaregression. *BMJ Open, 6,* e011827. https://doi.org/10.1136/bmjopen-2016-011827

Sobell, M.B., & Sobell, L.C. (2000). Stepped care as a heuristic approach to the treatment of alcohol problems. *Journal of Consulting and Clinical Psychology, 68*(4), 573–579. https://doi.org/10.1037/0022-006X.68.4.573

Spitzer, R.L., Kroenke, K., Williams, J.B.W., & Lowe, B. (2006). A brief measure for assessing generalized anxiety disorder: The GAD-7. *Archives of Internal Medicine, 166*(10), 1092–1097. https://doi.org/10.1001/archinte.166.10.1092

Substance Abuse and Mental Health Services Administration. (2020). *Treating substance use disorder in older adults. Treatment Improvement Protocol (TIP)* (Series No. 26, SAMHSA Publication No. PEP20-02-01-011).

Tampi, R., Chhatlani, A., Ahmad, H., Balaram, K., Dey, J., Escobar, R., & Lingamchetty, T. (2019). Pharmacotherapy for substance use disorders among older adults: A systematic review of randomized controlled trials. *American Journal of Geriatric Psychiatry, 27*(3), S161-S163. https://doi.org/10.1016/j.jagp.2019.01.072

Towers, A., Sheridan, J., Newcombe, D., & Szabó, Á. (2018). *New Zealanders' alcohol consumption patterns across the lifespan.* Health Promotion Agency.

US Department of Agriculture and US Department of Health and Human Services. (2020). *Dietary guidelines for americans, 2020-2025* (9th ed.). https://www.dietary-guidelines.gov/

van den Berg, J.F., Kok, R.M., van Marwijk, H.W.J., van der Mast, R.C., Naarding, P., Oude Voshaar, R.C., Stek, M.L., Verhaak, P.F.M., de Waal, M.W.M., & Comjis, H.C. (2014). Correlates of alcohol abstinence and at-risk alcohol consumption in older adults with depression: The NESDO study. *American Journal of Geriatric Psychiatry, 22*(9), 866-874. https://doi.org/10.1016/j.jagp.2013.04.006

Wetterling, T., Veltrup, C., John, U., & Driessen, M. (2003). Late onset alcoholism. *European Psychiatry, 18*(3), 112-118. https://doi.org/10.1016/S0924-9338(03)00025-7

Wild, B., Eckl, A., Herzog, W., Niehoff, D., Lechner, S., Maatouk, I., Schellberg, D., Brenner, H., Müller, H., & Löwe, B. (2014). Assessing Generalized Anxiety Disorder in elderly people using the GAD-7 and GAD-2 scales: Results of a validation study. *American Journal of Geriatric Psychiatry, 22*(10), 1029-1038. https://doi.org/10.1016/j.jagp.2013.01.076

Wolitzky-Taylor, K., Brown, L.A., Roy-Byrne, P., Sherbourne, C., Stein, M.B., Sullivan, G., Bystritsky, A., & Craske, M.G. (2015). The impact of alcohol use severity on anxiety treatment outcomes in a large effectiveness trial in primary care. *Journal of Anxiety Disorders, 30,* 88-93. https://doi.org/10.1016/j.janxdis.2014.12.011

World Health Organization. (2022). *Ageing and health.* https://www.who.int/news-room/fact-sheets/detail/ageing-and-health

Yang, J.C., Roman-Urrestarazu, A., & Brayne, C. (2018). Binge alcohol and substance use across birth cohorts and the global financial crisis in the United States. *PLOS ONE, 13*(6), e0199741. https://doi.org/10.1371/journal.pone.0199741

Zemore, S.E., Lui, C., Mericle, A., Hemberg, J., & Kaskutas, L.A. (2018). A longitudinal study of the comparative efficacy of Women for Sobriety, LifeRing, SMART Recovery, and 12-step groups for those with AUD. *Journal of Substance Abuse Treatment, 88,* 18-26. https://doi.org/10.1016/j.jsat.2018.02.004

Notes on Supplementary Materials

DOWNLOAD

The following materials for your book can be downloaded free of charge once you register on our website:

Appendix: Tools and Resources

Appendix 1: Patient Health Questionnaire-9 (PHQ-9)
Appendix 2: Generalized Anxiety Disorder Screener (GAD-7)
Appendix 3: Alcohol Use Disorders Identification Test – Consumption (AUDIT-C)
Appendix 4: Short Michigan Alcoholism Screening Test – Geriatric Version (SMAST-G)

How to proceed:

1. Create a user account (or, if you have already one, please log in)

For customers from the USA and Canada:
hgf.io/login-us

For customers from the rest of the world:
hgf.io/login-eu

2. Download your supplementary materials

Go to **My supplementary materials** in your account dashboard and enter the code below. You will automatically be redirected to the download area, where you can access and download the supplementary materials.

Code: **B-TM63M4**

To make sure you have permanent direct access to all the materials, we recommend that you download them and save them on your computer.

Patient Health Questionnaire-9 (PHQ-9)

The PHQ-9 is a recommended screener for older adults with depressive symptoms. Adapted from Kroenke and colleagues (2001).

	Not at all	Several days	More than half the days	Nearly every day
1. Little interest or pleasure in doing things	0	1	2	3
2. Feeling down, depressed, or hopeless	0	1	2	3
3. Trouble falling asleep or staying asleep, or sleeping too much	0	1	2	3
4. Feeling tired or having little energy	0	1	2	3
5. Poor appetite or overeating	0	1	2	3
6. Feeling bad about yourself – or that you are a failure or have let yourself or your family down	0	1	2	3
7. Trouble concentrating on things, such as in reading the newspaper or watching television	0	1	2	3
8. Moving or speaking so slowly that other people could have noticed. Or the opposite – being so fidgety or restless that you have been moving around a lot more than usual	0	1	2	3
9. Thoughts that you would be better off dead, or of hurting yourself	0	1	2	3
10. If you checked off any problems, how difficult have these problems made it for you to do your work, take care of things at home, or get along with other people?	Not difficult at all	Somewhat difficult	Very difficult	Extremely difficult

Scoring: Add up each column and sum the columns to calculate the total score. Use the scoring guide below to interpret the score. Diagnoses of major depressive disorder or other depressive disorder also require impairment of social, occupational, or other important areas of functioning (Question #10) and the ruling out normal bereavement, a history of a manic episode (bipolar disorder), and a physical disorder, medication, or other drug as the biological cause of the depressive symptoms.

See p. 103 for instructions on how to obtain the full-sized worksheets as printable PDFs.

Total score depression severity	Depression severity
1–4	Minimal depression
5–9	Mild depression
10–14	Moderate depression
15–19	Moderately severe depression

Note. Developed by Drs. Robert L. Spitzer, Janet B. W. Williams, Kurt Kroenke and colleagues, with an educational grant from Pfizer Inc. No permission required to reproduce, translate, display or distribute.

This page may be reproduced by the purchaser for personal/clinical use.
From: E. L. Woodhead: *Unhealthy Alcohol Use in Older Adults.* © 2024 Hogrefe Publishing
(978-0-88937-510-9) © 2024 Hogrefe Publishing

See p. 103 for instructions on how to obtain the full-sized worksheets as printable PDFs.

Generalized Anxiety Disorder Screener (GAD-7)

The GAD-7 can help to differentiate unhealthy alcohol use from anxiety disorders among older adults. Adapted from Spitzer and colleagues (2006).

Over the last 2 weeks, how often have you been bothered by the following problems?	Not at all	Several days	More than half the days	Nearly every day
1. Feeling nervous, anxious, or on edge	0	1	2	3
2. Not being able to stop or control worrying	0	1	2	3
3. Worrying too much about different things	0	1	2	3
4. Feeling tired or having little energy	0	1	2	3
5. Trouble relaxing	0	1	2	3
6. Being so restless that it is hard to sit still	0	1	2	3
7. Feeling afraid as if something awful might happen	0	1	2	3
ADD COLUMNS				
TOTAL SCORE				
8. If you checked off any problems, how difficult have these problems made it for you to do your work, take care of things at home, or get along with other people?	Not difficult at all	Some-what difficult	Very difficult	Extremely difficult

Scoring: 0–7 = no provisional diagnosis; 8+ = probable anxiety disorder.

Note. The GAD-7 is in the public domain. No permission required.

This page may be reproduced by the purchaser for personal/clinical use.
From: E. L. Woodhead: *Unhealthy Alcohol Use in Older Adults.* © 2024 Hogrefe Publishing
(978-0-88937-510-9) © 2024 Hogrefe Publishing

See p. 103 for instructions on how to obtain the full-sized worksheets as printable PDFs.

Alcohol Use Disorders Identification Test – Consumption (AUDIT-C)

The AUDIT-C has been translated into multiple languages and is used as a screener in SBIRT. Adapted from Bush and colleagues (1998).

1. How often did you have a drink containing alcohol in the past year?				
Never	Monthly or less	Two to four times a month	Two to three times per week	Four or more times a week
2. How many drinks containing alcohol did you have on a typical day when you were drinking, in the past year?				
1 or 2 drinks	3 or 4	5 or 6	7 to 9	10 or more
3. How often did you have six or more drinks on one occasion in the past year?				
Never	Less than monthly	Monthly	Weekly	Daily or almost daily

Scoring: In men, a score of 4 or more is considered positive; in women, a score of 3 or more is considered positive.

Note. The AUDIT-C is a modified version of the 10-item Alcohol Use Disorders Identification Test developed by the World Health Organization and published in 1998. The AUDIT-C is available for use in the public domain. No permission required.

This page may be reproduced by the purchaser for personal/clinical use.
From: E. L. Woodhead: *Unhealthy Alcohol Use in Older Adults.* © 2024 Hogrefe Publishing (978-0-88937-510-9) © 2024 Hogrefe Publishing

See p. 103 for instructions on how to obtain the full-sized worksheets as printable PDFs.

Short Michigan Alcoholism Screening Test – Geriatric Version (SMAST-G)

The SMAST-G is the only alcohol assessment designed specifically for older adults, and it is reliable and valid in this population. Adapted from Blow and colleagues (1991).

Please answer yes or no to the following questions:	Yes	No
1. When talking with others, do you ever underestimate how much you drink?		
2. After a few drinks, have you sometimes not eaten or been able to skip a meal because you did not feel hungry?		
3. Does having a few drinks help decrease your shakiness or tremors?		
4. Does alcohol sometimes make it hard for you to remember parts of the day or night?		
5. Do you usually take a drink to calm your nerves?		
6. Do you drink to take your mind off problems?		
7. Have you ever increased your drinking after experiencing a loss in your life?		
8. Has a doctor or nurse ever said they were worried or concerned about your drinking?		
9. Have you ever made rules to manage your drinking?		
10. When you feel lonely, does having a drink help?		
Scoring: Score 1 point for each yes answer and total the responses; 2 or more points are indicative of an alcohol problem. The extra question below should not be calculated in the final score but should be asked, for additional information.		
Extra question: Do you drink alcohol and take mood- or mind-altering drugs, including prescription tranquilizers, prescription sleeping pills, prescription pain pills, or any illicit drugs?		
Note. Reprinted with permission from "The Michigan Alcoholism Screening Test-Geriatric Version (MAST-G): A new elderly specific screening instrument" by F. C. Blow and colleagues. © 1991 by The Regents of the University of Michigan.		

This page may be reproduced by the purchaser for personal/clinical use.
From: E. L. Woodhead: *Unhealthy Alcohol Use in Older Adults*. © 2024 Hogrefe Publishing (978-0-88937-510-9) © 2024 Hogrefe Publishing

See p. 103 for instructions on how to obtain the full-sized worksheets as printable PDFs.

Get the science on helping reduce stress in family caregivers of people with dementia

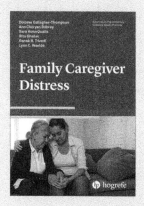

Dolores Gallagher-Thompson / Ann Choryan Bilbrey / Sara Honn Qualls / Rita Ghatak / Ranak B. Trivedi / Lynn C. Waelde

Family Caregiver Distress
2023, xii + 100 pp.,
$29.80 / € 24.95
ISBN 978-0-88937-517-8
Also available as eBook

This is the first book that takes a "deep dive" to answer the questions that mental health providers encounter when working with family caregivers. Just what are the unique issues family caregivers face? How does this impact their mental health? What can providers do to help?

Based on research and clinical experiences of the authors, this volume in our *Advances in Psychotherapy* series focuses on examining the specific issues that caregivers of people with Alzheimer's disease or other forms of dementia face. Practitioners learn about the best tools for assessment and which evidence-based interventions help reduce caregiver distress – including cognitive behavioral therapy, acceptance and commitment therapy, and mindfulness and multicomponent intervention programs.

Resources in the appendix include a caretaker intake interview, and the book is interspersed with clinical vignettes that highlight issues of diversity, equity, and inclusion – making this an essential text for mental health providers from a variety of disciplines including psychology, psychiatry, nursing, social work, marriage and family counseling, as well as trainees in these disciplines.

www.hogrefe.com

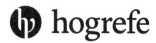

Expert guidance on working psychologically with older adults

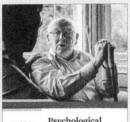

Nancy A. Pachana / Victor Molinari / Larry W. Thompson / Dolores Gallagher-Thompson (Eds.)

Psychological Assessment and Treatment of Older Adults

2021, viii + 250 pp.,
$59.00 / € 50.95
ISBN 978-0-88937-571-0
Also available as eBook

Mental health practitioners are encountering an ever-growing number of older adults and so an up-to-date and comprehensive text addressing the special considerations that arise in the psychological assessment and treatment of this population is vital.

This accessible handbook does just that by introducing the key topics that psychologists and other health professionals face when working with older adults. Each area is introduced and then the special considerations for older adults are explored, including specific ethical and healthcare system issues. The use of case examples brings the topics further to life. An important feature of the book is the interweaving of diversity issues (culture, race, sexuality, etc.) within the text to lend an inclusive, contemporary insight into these important practice components. The Pikes Peak Geropsychology Knowledge and Skill Assessment Tool is included in an appendix so readers can test their knowledge, which will be helpful for those aiming for board certification in geropsychology (ABGERO).

This an ideal text for mental health professionals transitioning to work with older clients, for those wanting to improve their knowledge for their regular practice, and for trainees or young clinicians just starting out.

www.hogrefe.com

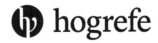